Primary Care for Emergency Physicians

Bobby K. Desai • Alpa Desai
Latha Ganti • Samyr Elbadri
Editors

Primary Care for Emergency Physicians

Second Edition

Springer

Editors
Bobby K. Desai
College of Medicine
University of Central Florida
Ocala, FL, USA

Alpa Desai
Community Health and Family Medicine
University of Florida
Gainesville, FL, USA

Latha Ganti
College of Medicine
University of Central Florida
Orlando, FL, USA

Samyr Elbadri
College of Medicine Department
of Emergency Medicine
University of Central Florida
Orlando, FL, USA

ISBN 978-3-031-64675-1 ISBN 978-3-031-64676-8 (eBook)
https://doi.org/10.1007/978-3-031-64676-8

This Springer imprint is published by the registered company Springer Nature Switzerland AG
The registered company address is: Gewerbestrasse 11, 6330 Cham, Switzerland

Preface

While primary care and emergency care may initially appear to be on opposite ends of the overall spectrum of care of a patient, these specialties also do have areas of overlap. An emergency physician's primary role is to manage true emergencies; however, many patients present to the emergency department due to lack of primary care access and require urgent, rather than emergent, treatment. Many emergency physicians lack training in primary care disease processes. We hope this book helps to improve their comfort level in treatment of these conditions. Emergency physicians can do the patient a great service by evaluating outpatient disease processes patients may present with and initiating appropriate therapy, with a discharge plan to follow up with their primary care physician.

Contents

Contributors

Graham Clifford Department of Emergency Medicine, University of Florida College of Medicine, Gainesville, FL, USA

Alpa Desai Department of Community Health and Family Medicine, University of Florida College of Medicine, Gainesville, FL, USA

Samuel Dickmann Department of Community Health and Family Medicine, University of Florida College of Medicine, Gainesville, FL, USA

Shane Dluzneski University of Central Florida, Orlando, FL, USA

Run Gan Department of Community Health and Family Medicine, University of Florida College of Medicine, Gainesville, FL, USA

Karyn Governale Department of Community Health and Family Medicine, UF Health Shands Hospital, Gainesville, FL, USA

Derrick Huang University of Central Florida, Orlando, FL, USA

Charles Hwang Department of Emergency Medicine, University of Florida College of Medicine, Gainesville, FL, USA

Elisabeth H. W. Hwang Department of Emergency Medicine, University of Florida College of Medicine, Gainesville, FL, USA

Harman Kaur Division of Pediatric Emergency Medicine, Arnold Palmer Hospital For Children, Orlando, FL, USA

Morgan Killian University of Central Florida, Orlando, FL, USA

Emily Macauley University of Central Florida, Orlando, FL, USA

James Medley Department of Community Health and Family Medicine, University of Florida College of Medicine, Gainesville, FL, USA

Bryson Renouard Texas A&M University, College Station, TX, USA

Dipal Shah University of Central Florida, Orlando, FL, USA

Michael Seth Smith Division of Sports Medicine, Department of Orthopedics and Rehabilitation, University of Florida, Gainesville, FL, USA

Sakina Sojar Division of Pediatric Emergency Medicine, Warren Alpert Medical School of Brown University, Providence, RI, USA

Department of Emergency Medicine, University of Florida College of Medicine, Gainesville, FL, USA

Brooke Taylor University of Central Florida, Orlando, FL, USA

Josh Walker University of Central Florida, Orlando, FL, USA

Christopher Wallace University of Central Florida, Orlando, FL, USA

Rohan Wanchu University of Central Florida, Orlando, FL, USA

Emily Weeks University of Central Florida, Orlando, FL, USA

James Link Wilson University of Central Florida, Orlando, FL, USA

Mar'Tina Wimberly Department of Community Health and Family Medicine, University of Florida College of Medicine, Gainesville, FL, USA

Lucas Winter University of Central Florida, Orlando, FL, USA

1 Headache

Samuel Dickmann

1.1 Introduction

Headache remains a common cause of presentation to the emergency department (ED) worldwide, estimated at 1–4% of total visits, and around 3–5% of patients in the USA will seek care in the ED for a headache on at least one occasion [1–3]. There are many possible causes of headaches, including several severe or life-threatening causes, which creates a challenge for clinicians, particularly with the potentially severe consequences of a misdiagnosis. Thankfully, most cases do not stem from life-threatening causes, and a methodical approach to the evaluation simplifies the diagnosis and general treatment options. Further, the initial steps of outpatient management for primary headaches can easily be initiated in the ED, facilitating the transition of care from ED clinicians to a patient's primary care clinician (PCC) or neurologist.

1.2 Classification and Differential Diagnosis

Per the International Headache Society (IHS) classification system, headaches are divided into two broad classes: primary and secondary [4]. In primary headache, the headache itself is the pathologic condition, while secondary headaches exist as one of possibly many symptoms with an underlying causative pathology.

Broadly, the three major primary headaches are tension-type headache, migraine (with or without aura), and cluster headache (the most common member of the trigeminal autonomic cephalalgias) [4]. Many less common primary headaches have been defined, including primary cough headache, primary headache associated with sexual activity, hypnic (sleep) headache, and benign thunderclap headache. These

S. Dickmann (✉)
Department of Community Health and Family Medicine, University of Florida College of Medicine, Gainesville, FL, USA

B. K. Desai et al. (eds.), *Primary Care for Emergency Physicians*,
https://doi.org/10.1007/978-3-031-64676-8_1

headaches must fulfill specific criteria, must exist in the absence of an underlying causative condition, and are generally diagnoses of exclusion. The nuance of these headaches would be better managed by a patient's primary care clinician (PCC) or a neurologist and is beyond the scope of our discussion here. Features of the three main primary headaches are further described in Table 1.1, derived from the International Classification of Headache Disorders, third edition (ICHD-3).

Specific note should be made regarding a migraine aura. The aura is a transient and fully resolving neurologic phenomenon, developing gradually over about 5 min, lasting less than 1 h, and often preceded by a prodrome of vague symptoms, such as depression, irritability, yawning, food cravings, or neck stiffness [4, 5]. Some patients can predict the onset of their headaches because of a predictable prodrome and aura. The aura itself manifests with positive and negative symptoms involving the visual, auditory, somatosensory, and motor systems. Positive symptoms may include flashing lights in vision, visualization of irregular shapes, increased tinnitus, hearing unusual noises, and dysesthesias or jerking in extremities. Negative symptoms might include visual loss, decreased hearing, or loss of sensation in an extremity. Importantly, these features are predictable, fully resolve in a fairly short time, and precede or immediately accompany the headache [4, 5].

Table 1.1 Primary headaches

Category	Tension-type headache	Migraine headache	Cluster headache
Location	Bilateral, often posterior (but may be bitemporal)	Unilateral, sometimes becoming bilateral, often in the frontal or temporal region	Always unilateral, orbital, and periorbital
Nature	Aching, dull, waxing and waning	Throbbing, pounding, dull, aching, pulsating, gradual onset over 1–2 h	Deep, continuous, stabbing or "ice pick," rapid onset
Severity	Mild to moderate	Moderate to severe	Severe
Duration	From hours to days Often recurring multiple days consecutively	Typically 4–72 h	Episodic, occurring multiple times in a short period, then remitting for weeks to months Headaches last from minutes to hours, up to eight times a day
Associated symptoms	Neck stiffness	Nausea, photophobia, phonophobia, +/− aura	Unilateral autonomic symptoms • Tearing • Rhinorrhea • Ptosis • Meiosis
Other features	Often able to continue activities through the headache Pain tends to be worse later in the day	Unable to continue activities through the headache—need to lie down and rest May wake from sleep with headache Female predominance: 3:1	Rapidly responsive to 100% inhaled oxygen Male predominance

Secondary headaches are highly varied, owing to the numerous underlying conditions that manifest with headache as a symptom. Secondary headaches encompass a variety of benign and self-limited conditions (such as caffeine withdrawal headaches) to severe and life-threatening conditions (subarachnoid hemorrhage, primary CNS or metastatic neoplasm). An exhaustive review of diagnostic criteria is simply impractical—interested clinicians should refer to the ICHD-3. Instead, clinicians should keep in mind a general classification system for secondary headaches, focusing on each element in turn as a possible source of headache. Table 1.2 lists secondary headaches by categories.

Table 1.2 Secondary headaches

Categories	Specific conditions and details
Trauma or injury to the head and/or neck	• Mild traumatic brain injury (concussion) • Moderate to severe traumatic brain injury • Whiplash • Cranial or cervical fracture • Craniotomy
Cranial or cervical vascular disorder • Ischemia and thrombosis • Hemorrhage • Malformation • Dissection • Arteritis	• Ischemia and thrombosis – Ischemic cerebrovascular accident (CVA) – Transient ischemic attack (TIA) – Cerebral venous thrombosis • Intracranial hemorrhage – Epidural hemorrhage – Subdural hemorrhage (SDH) – Subarachnoid hemorrhage (ruptured intracranial aneurysm) – Intracerebral hemorrhage (hemorrhagic CVA) • Vascular malformation – Intracranial aneurysm (unruptured) – Arteriovenous malformation • Intracranial or cervical artery dissection • Arteritis (e.g., giant cell arteritis)
Nonvascular intracranial disorder • Increased CSF pressure • Decreased CSF pressure • Neoplasms • Noninfectious inflammation • Seizure	• Increased CSF pressure—positional headache, better when erect – Idiopathic intracranial hypertension (pseudotumor cerebri) • Decreased CSF pressure—positional headache, better when recumbent – Post-lumbar puncture headache – CSF fistula • Intracranial neoplasms—either CNS primary or as a site of metastasis • Noninfectious inflammatory disease – Neurosarcoidosis – Aseptic meningitis – Noninfectious inflammatory intracranial disease (SLE, Behcet's syndrome, ADEM) • Epileptic seizure (ictal or postictal headache) • Chiari malformation (type 1)—cervical pain and suboccipital headache provoked by exertion or cough

(continued)

Table 1.2 (continued)

Categories	Specific conditions and details
Medications and substances—exposure, overexposure, and withdrawal	• Medication use: phosphodiesterase inhibitors (Viagra, Cialis), nitroglycerin, nifedipine and nimodipine, digitalis, disulfiram, hydralazine, imipramine • Medication overuse: opioids, triptans, NSAIDs and acetaminophen, aspirin, CGRP antagonists • Substances: caffeine, nicotine, alcohol, cocaine, cannabis, carbon monoxide, other toxic exposures
Disorder of the cranium and other structures • Cranial bones • Eyes • Nose or paranasal sinuses • TMJ	• Cranial bone destruction (multiple myeloma, Paget's disease) • Eyes – Acute angle-closure glaucoma – Ocular inflammatory disorder (uveitis) – Chronic refractive error • Nose or paranasal sinuses (allergic rhinosinusitis, chronic sinusitis) • Temporomandibular joint dysfunction
Infectious	• Intracranial infection (bacterial meningitis, herpes encephalitis) • Cranial and extracranial infection (mastoiditis, cranial osteomyelitis, acute rhinosinusitis, acute otitis media) • Systemic infection (e.g., influenza, HIV/AIDS, COVID-19)
Disordered homeostasis • Hypoxia or hypercapnia • Dialysis • Arterial hypertension • Others	• Hypoxia or hypercapnia – High altitude exposure – Diving – Sleep apnea and obesity hypoventilation syndrome • Dialysis headache • Arterial hypertension – Hypertensive crisis (SBP ≥180 mmHg, DBP ≥120 mmHg)—may have encephalopathy present – Eclampsia/preeclampsia • Hypothyroidism, fasting, dehydration
Psychiatric	• Somatization disorder • Worsening of headache due to undertreated mood disorder (e.g., generalized anxiety disorder, major depressive disorder)

1.3 Pathophysiology

The pathophysiology of headaches is complex and varied. Lacking intrinsic pain receptors, the brain tissue itself is not the source of acute headache pain. Rather, headaches are primarily caused by inflammation and pressure changes at the vasculature or the meninges, as in subarachnoid hemorrhage or bacterial meningitis, for instance, or by activation of peripheral myofascial nociceptors, as in tension-type headaches or a cervical fracture.

Migraine headaches are a particularly complex and poorly understood phenomenon, attributed to a primary neuronal dysfunction [5] initiating a sequence of neurological depolarization (known as cortical spreading depression) [6], alterations in blood–brain barrier permeability, and activation of trigeminal afferents [5, 7].

In chronic headache disorders generally, sensitization of pain pathways in the central nervous system (CNS) is believed to play an increasing role over time, as chronic nociceptive input triggers changes that induce central sensitization and an upregulation of potentially painful stimuli [8]. This pathophysiology makes the management of chronic headache potentially complicated and difficult.

1.4 Epidemiology

The epidemiology for patients presenting with acute headache to a specific emergency department (ED) cannot be known without studying that location specifically, but studies have suggested that primary headaches account for between 45 and 60% of headache cases in ED environments worldwide [1–3, 9]. Secondary headaches are less common, in the range of 20–30%, and headaches that cannot be easily classified make up a significantly smaller portion, having features of both primary and secondary headaches [1–3, 9].

Of primary headaches, migraine is the one most commonly encountered by clinicians [1, 2, 9], likely due to the severity and debility, though tension-type headaches are the most common of the primary headaches overall [5]. Owing to the lesser severity and the ability to continue activities through the headache, many patients will manage tension-type headaches with over-the-counter remedies and will not present to a clinician for evaluation. Cluster headaches are of low incidence generally (<1%), but during episodes almost all patients will seek medical attention, due to the severity of the headache.

Regarding secondary headaches, epidemiologic data is somewhat limited and inconsistent, possibly due to inconsistent usage of diagnostic criteria. Sinusitis, viral syndromes, uncontrolled hypertension, and cervical myofascial pain are all major causes, while SAH and intracranial bleeding typically make up between 0.5 and 2% of overall headache presentations [2, 3, 9]. Infectious meningitis was around 0.5% of overall presentations in one study [2]. Life-threatening secondary headaches of all causes make up a minority of presentations, between 2 and 15% of ED presentations for headache worldwide [2, 3, 9]. Thus, the vast majority of headaches seen in emergency departments are not considered life-threatening.

1.5 Evaluation

To evaluate a patient presenting to the ED with acute headache, start with an appropriate differential diagnosis. Knowing that primary headaches are statistically the most likely, a wise clinician would have a high suspicion for a primary headache when evaluating patients. The best approach is to ask pointed questions, trying to exclude secondary headaches and particularly life-threatening ones. If necessary, proceed by using diagnostic criteria to determine the type of primary headache present, but if life-threatening and serious causes can be safely excluded and the diagnosis is uncertain, it would be reasonable to defer diagnosis to a patient's PCC or neurologist and simply list "primary headache disorder" or "undifferentiated benign headache" in communications.

Consider the utility of each evaluation element in guiding a differential diagnosis. An excellent clinician considers each history question and each physical exam maneuver as a diagnostic tool, increasing the positive or negative likelihood of a specific diagnosis. Asking a patient in the ED, "Is this the worst headache of your life?" is unlikely to be helpful. In this author's experience of clinic and hospital settings, a high number of patients will always answer affirmatively. Rather, ask, "When was the last time you had a headache like this?" or "Have you had this type of headache before?" Patients who describe prior similar headaches are more likely to have a primary headache disorder.

Proceed by collecting the basic features of the headache (e.g., location, severity, nature, aggravating and alleviating factors, and associated symptoms) and then evaluate for specific symptoms of or risk factors for secondary headaches. Certain historical features are more suggestive of secondary headaches, as detailed in Table 1.3.

Details such as the presence of a fever, present URI symptoms, meningeal symptoms (such as severe neck stiffness), focal and persistent neurologic symptoms (weakness, numbness, dysarthria, aphasia), or a distinctly positional nature of the headache (worse when lying down or worse when sitting up) make a secondary

Table 1.3 Historical features suggesting a high-risk or secondary headache [10, 11]

High-risk features
• Sudden-onset headache (severe, persistent headache reaching maximal intensity within less than 1–2 min) suggests subarachnoid hemorrhage, arterial dissection, venous sinus thrombosis, or other severe or life-threatening cause
• No similar headaches in the past (e.g., "first" or "worst" headache) suggest intracranial hemorrhage or CNS infection or a space-occupying lesion
• Concomitant infection (such as sinusitis, otitis media, pharyngitis) suggests meningitis or intracranial abscess
• Altered mental status or an associated seizure suggests significant intracranial pathology
• Persistent visual impairment suggests acute angle-closure glaucoma, temporal arteritis, or idiopathic intracranial hypertension
• Rapid headache associated with exertion raises the possibility of carotid artery dissection, reversible cerebral vasoconstriction, or intracranial hemorrhage
• Age over 50 increases the likelihood of a secondary headache
• Immunosuppression (from immunotherapy or due to HIV/AIDS) increases the likelihood of atypical infections and malignancy
• Persistent visual disturbance suggests acute angle-closure glaucoma, temporal arteritis or optic nerve ischemia, idiopathic intracranial hypertension, or PRES
• Persistent focal neurologic deficits suggest an intracranial mass lesion or ischemia
• Pregnancy or recent postpartum state raises the possibility of preeclampsia, particularly, and thrombosis in general
• Anticoagulant use significantly increases the likelihood of intracranial hemorrhage; aspirin and NSAIDs also increase risk
• Acute headaches among multiple close associates (family members, coworkers) suggest carbon monoxide poisoning or other toxic exposure

headache much more likely. Additional features such as sudden and abrupt onset of a severe headache, any history of recent head trauma, lack or any prior similar headaches, or age over 50 years old increase the likelihood of secondary headaches [10, 11].

The physical exam should be guided by the history, performing appropriate maneuvers that help to hone and limit the differential diagnosis. Start with an assessment of the vital signs, particularly focusing on the temperature, blood pressure, and oxygen saturation as most likely to be helpful in evaluating a patient with acute headache.

A neurologic exam is necessary for all patients, as "abnormal results from neurologic examination are the best clinical parameters to predict structural intracranial pathology" [12]. Many signs can be evaluated briefly through simple conversation with the patient, including orientation, recent and remote memory, and speech. Evaluate the cranial nerves, particularly pupillary reflexes and visual fields, facial sensation and facial muscle movement, tongue protrusion and palatal elevation, and shoulder shrug strength. Follow this with examination of strength in the upper and lower extremities and sensation using light touch in all extremities. Evaluation of reflexes should include the biceps, triceps, brachioradialis, patellar and Achilles tendons, and the plantar reflex. Finger-to-nose and heel-to-shin testing completes a basic neurologic exam.

Further physical exam should be guided by the differential diagnosis. For the examination of head, eyes, ears, nose, and throat (HEENT), perform a fundoscopic exam when considering diagnoses that would increase intracranial pressure. Examining for signs of cranial trauma is important when considering intracranial hemorrhage or concussion. Temporal artery tenderness or diminished pulse suggests temporal arteritis. Mastoid tenderness suggests possible mastoiditis when found in a patient with acute otitis media or acute sinusitis. Pain with direct pressure on the frontal or maxillary sinuses near the nose suggests acute bacterial sinusitis.

Otherwise, a neck exam of flexion, extension, and rotation to assess for meningismus (which would increase the likelihood of meningitis or SAH) can be performed quickly. Briefly looking at the skin of patients can indicate pallor, diaphoresis, or bruising that would guide the differential. A full psychiatric evaluation is impractical in the ED, and it would be reasonable to defer this to the patient's PCC once life-threatening causes of headache have been ruled out. High-risk features are detailed in Table 1.4.

The decision to order labs or imaging should be guided by the differential diagnosis, seeking to clarify any areas of uncertainty. For primary headaches, further tests are generally unnecessary, so consider labs or imaging when secondary headaches are high on the differential. In fact, multiple guidelines discourage any CNS imaging for patients with low-risk clinical features [13]. Patients with a new, severe, nontraumatic headache reaching maximum intensity within 1 h should be considered via the Ottawa Subarachnoid Hemorrhage Rule (see Table 1.5). Guidelines regarding specific imaging modalities when assessing for specific life-threatening conditions can be found in Table 1.7 of the chapter appendix.

Table 1.4 Physical exam signs suggesting a high-risk or secondary headache [11]

High-risk signs
• Abnormal vital signs—fever, severe hypertension, hypoxia • Toxic appearance—lethargy, pallor, diaphoresis • Decreased level of consciousness—obtundation, confusion • Neurologic abnormalities—any *new* focal or non-focal, *persistent* neurologic abnormality – This is the single best predictor of serious intracranial pathology [12] – Migraines can present with focal neurologic abnormalities, but these should be consistent with the patient's prior migraine symptoms. Often, these are positive symptoms. (See above regarding negative and positive symptoms of migraine aura.) • Meningismus • Ophthalmologic findings—papilledema, retinal hemorrhage, visual field deficits, increased intraocular pressure, sluggish pupillary response

Table 1.5 Ottawa Subarachnoid Hemorrhage Rule [10, 13]

Consider imaging if *any* of the following features are present
• Symptoms of neck pain or stiffness • Age ≥40 years old • Witnessed loss of consciousness • Onset during exertion • Thunderclap headache (peak intensity almost immediately) • Limited neck flexion on exam

Laboratory testing is generally not indicated in the workup of acute nontraumatic headache, except when investigating specific secondary headaches. For example, in an older individual, a normal ESR greatly diminishes the likelihood of temporal arteritis. Lumbar puncture and CSF analysis should be considered if subarachnoid hemorrhage is suspected even after a negative head CT or if meningitis or encephalitis is suspected. In the latter situation, analyses should include a cell count, gram stain, protein and glucose measurement, and CSF culture. In combination with a negative head CT, absence of RBCs and absence of xanthochromia on CSF analysis rule out a SAH [13]. If idiopathic intracranial hypertension or cryptococcal meningitis is suspected, an opening pressure should be measured.

1.6 Treatment

Prior to any discussion of treatment, one major caveat is critical: a positive response to analgesia does not predict headache etiology, and empiric treatment should not be used to aid diagnosis [14]. Even the severe headache of subarachnoid hemorrhage may respond positively to a typical migraine cocktail [14].

Starting with primary headache disorders, treatment options are varied and typically fall into acute (abortive) and chronic (preventive) categories. Chronic treatment for primary headache disorders should be administered through the patient's PCC or neurologist. Preventative therapy for migraines, such as with daily topiramate, propranolol, or a calcitonin gene-related peptide (CGRP) antagonist, can be highly effective but requires a long-term patient-clinician relationship for appropriate monitoring. ED clinicians should focus on acute treatment in the ED setting followed by an efficient transfer of care back to the patient's community clinicians.

Acute treatment of severe migraine is the statistically most-likely concern for ED clinicians. Generally, for mild migraine headaches, NSAIDs are first-line therapy and quite effective, but more severe migraines require a combination of agents for effective therapy. Triptans are first-line therapy for moderate to severe migraines, and they are very effective overall [15]. Coadministration of a triptan with an NSAID has shown greater efficacy than triptans alone [16]. CGRP antagonists have shown efficacy acutely, particularly as salvage therapy for patients who have not responded to triptans [17], and ergotamines are typically reserved for patients with severe and refractory migraines or status migrainosus. Parenteral dexamethasone has shown significant efficacy in preventing headache recurrence in the short term (24–72 h) [18], so consider giving dexamethasone along with triptan or CGRP therapy for severe migraines. In general, guidelines encourage clinicians to avoid opioids for treatment of acute headaches [19]. Details of individual agents, dosing, risks, and side effects for various agents can be found in Table 1.6.

Table 1.6 Pharmacologic treatment of headaches

Category	Mechanism	Dosing	Comments and risks
NSAIDs, acetaminophen, aspirin	Block the inflammatory arachidonic acid cascade at COX-1 and COX-2 to inhibit prostaglandin synthesis	• Ibuprofen 400–600 mg PO • Naproxen 220–500 mg PO • Acetaminophen 500–1000 mg PO or IV • Aspirin 500–1000 mg PO • Ketorolac 30 mg IV or 60 mg IM • Indomethacin 25–75 mg PO or IV	Adverse reactions for NSAIDs include gastric irritation, GI bleeding, and renal dysfunction. Aspirin causes permanent dysfunction of circulating platelets. Acetaminophen should be avoided in conjunction with ethanol and should be limited to no more than 3 g daily. Ibuprofen has a black box association with cardiovascular disease
Neuroleptics, antiemetics, antihistamines	Multiple pharmacologic targets, including dopaminergic blockade, acetylcholine sensitization	• Metoclopramide 10 mg IV • Prochlorperazine 10 mg IV or IM • Chlorpromazine 0.1 mg/kg slow IV infusion (1 mg/min); max dose 25 mg	These agents also have many possible adverse reactions, notably akathisia and dystonic reactions, sedation, and QTc prolongation. Clinicians are advised to familiarize themselves with the preferred agents. Side effects may be decreased or eliminated by pretreatment with diphenhydramine 12.5–25 mg IV

(continued)

Table 1.6 (continued)

Category	Mechanism	Dosing	Comments and risks
Triptans and DHE	Causes vasoconstriction via selective serotonergic agonism (5HT-1 for triptans, 5HT-1D for DHE)	• Sumatriptan 100 mg PO, 6 mg SC, 20 mg intranasal • Zolmitriptan 5 mg intranasal • Dihydroergotamine (DHE) 1 mg SC, IM, or IV Triptan dose can be repeated once, safely	These classes may contribute to serotonin syndrome, chest pain, and possibly coronary vasoconstriction. Avoid for patients with a history of Prinzmetal's angina, cardiovascular or cerebrovascular disease, uncontrolled hypertension, or concurrent MAOI or other vasoconstrictive medication use. Do not give triptans within 24 h of dihydroergotamine. DHE carries a black box warning for peripheral ischemia and cerebral vasospasm when given with 3A4 inhibitors (including macrolide antibiotics and protease inhibitors) and should not be used in hemiplegic or basilar migraine
Corticosteroids	Multiple anti-inflammatory, glucocorticoid, and mineralocorticoid effects	• Prednisone 60 mg PO • Methylprednisolone 125 mg IV • Dexamethasone 10–24 mg IV	Usually well tolerated as short-term therapy, but efficacy data are mixed regarding acute treatment. Primarily, corticosteroids have shown benefit in preventing migraine recurrence in the short term Note: daily steroid therapy should be initiated immediately if temporal arteritis is suspected
Calcitonin gene-related peptide (CGRP) antagonists	Antagonism at the calcitonin gene-related peptide receptor, mediating trigeminovascular pain transmission	• Rimegepant 75 mg PO • Ubrogepant 50–100 mg PO, may repeat in 2 h, max dose 200 mg/24 h • Zavegepant 10 mg intranasally	Can be highly effective, particularly if given in the early phase of migraine attacks. Should be avoided in pregnant patients and those with recent cardiovascular or cerebrovascular ischemic events

(continued)

Table 1.6 (continued)

Category	Mechanism	Dosing	Comments and risks
Opioids	Antagonism at opioid receptors	• Hydrocodone 5 mg or oxycodone 5 mg PO • Hydromorphone 0.5–1 mg IV	Opiates are pro-inflammatory and increase vasodilation, which is counterproductive in treatment of acute migraine. If opioids are the only medications by which the patient obtains relief, the physician should consider medication-overuse headache or opioid dependence as a cause. Consider usage in the very elderly or pregnant women where other agents are contraindicated or problematic

For tension-type headaches, data is somewhat lacking, but acute treatment for severe cases involves parenteral NSAIDs or antiemetics. Typical agents would include ketorolac (Toradol), metoclopramide, and chlorpromazine. In a systematic review, combination metoclopramide and diphenhydramine was superior to ketorolac [20].

For cluster headache, acute treatment is typically 100% pure oxygen (12 L/min) for 15 min [21] and administration of a triptan [22]. Verapamil is first line for prevention of cluster headache, and corticosteroids can also be used for prevention. Preventative therapy should likely be deferred to the patient's PCC or neurologist, where routine follow-up for dose titration and adverse effects can be accomplished.

For the undifferentiated headache, evidence-based guidelines are lacking, but available evidence suggests that treatments for acute migraine provide some relief in patients with undifferentiated headache. For instance, sumatriptan was effective for undifferentiated headache [23], and NSAIDs in combination with dopamine antagonists have also been effective therapy [24].

Appendix

Table 1.7 Dangerous causes of secondary headache

Diagnosis	Clinical features	Diagnostic testing	Interventions	Additional comments
Subarachnoid hemorrhage (SAH)	Severe, sudden-onset headache Different from other headaches	CT head Lumbar puncture	Neurosurgical consultation Blood pressure control Nimodipine Ventriculostomy	CT has extremely high sensitivity in the first 6 h, and then sensitivity steadily decreases Consider other causes of thunderclap headache
Cervical artery dissection (CeAD), internal carotid artery dissection (ICAD), or vertebral artery dissection (VAD)	New-onset head, neck, or facial pain ICAD: anterior circulation ischemia, Horner syndrome, cranial nerve abnormalities, or monocular vision loss VAD: posterior circulation ischemia	CT head/neck angiography	Anticoagulation vs antiplatelet therapy Consider thrombolytics in early ischemic stroke and extracranial dissection	Neurologic symptoms can be delayed after headache onset Rule out concomitant SAH before initiating anticoagulation Traumatic mechanism in 40%
Giant cell arteritis (GCA)	Headache in age >50 Polymyalgia rheumatica association Temporal artery abnormalities on examination Jaw claudication Visual loss (mainly monocular) Fevers	ESR (cannot rule out if normal) Temporal artery biopsy	Systemic glucocorticoid therapy	When suspicion is high, start steroid therapy while awaiting ESR/biopsy results Consider GCA and perform thorough scalp and ophthalmologic examination in elderly patients with fever of unknown source
Cerebral venous thrombosis (CVT)	Headache + signs of increased ICP or focal neurologic deficits	CT or MR venogram	Anticoagulation Endovascular thrombectomy if progressive symptoms despite anticoagulation	Highest risk if history of recent oral contraceptive use, pregnancy/ postpartum, thrombophilia

(continued)

Table 1.7 (continued)

Diagnosis	Clinical features	Diagnostic testing	Interventions	Additional comments
Idiopathic intracranial hypertension (IIH)	Most common in young, obese women in third or fourth decade of life Headache, vision loss, papilledema, transient visual obscurations (TVO), pulsatile tinnitus	Neuroimaging to rule out other space-occupying lesions Lumbar puncture with opening pressure >20 mmHg	Weight loss acetazolamide or furosemide optic nerve fenestration or CNS shunt if progressive vision loss	Cranial VI (abducens) palsy in at-risk patient population is suggestive Treat to prevent visual loss in 25% of patients
Acute angle-closure glaucoma (AACG)	Acute-onset monocular pain, headache, redness, decreased vision ± nausea vomiting Mid-fixed dilated pupil, "steamy cornea"	Ocular pressure >21 mmHg (most often >30 mmHg)	Ophthalmologic consultation Pressure-lowering eye drops Systemic osmotic therapy	Perform an eye examination on alert patients with dilated pupil and sudden-onset severe headache (can mimic SAH with PCOM aneurysm)
Bacterial meningitis	Fever, headache, altered mental status, nuchal rigidity	Lumbar puncture (+/− CT head) (see 2008 ACEP Clinical Policy on Acute Headache)	IV antibiotics Consider IV dexamethasone	Jolt accentuation, Brudzinski sign, Kernig sign, and nuchal rigidity: all are poorly sensitive physical examination findings
Preeclampsia	Headache in pregnancy >20 ± visual symptoms, abdominal pain, chest pain, shortness of breath, vomiting	SBP >140 mmHg or DBP >110 on two occasions + any of the following: proteinuria, thrombocytopenia, renal insufficiency, impaired liver function, pulmonary edema, cerebral or visual disturbances	Obstetric consultation Urgent delivery if severe symptoms Blood pressure management IV magnesium	Must consider diagnosis up to 6 weeks postpartum, highest risk in the first week postdelivery
Pituitary apoplexy	Severe headache Visual complaints, vomiting +/− Hypopituitarism	CT head noncontrast for hemorrhage MRI for pituitary mass	Neurosurgical consultation Systemic glucocorticoids for any adrenal insufficiency	Ocular paresis can occur, affecting CN III, IV, or VI (most commonly CN III)

(continued)

Table 1.7 (continued)

Diagnosis	Clinical features	Diagnostic testing	Interventions	Additional comments
Carbon monoxide poisoning	Flulike illness; worse each morning Mild: headache, nausea, myalgia, dizzy Severe: confusion, syncope, neurologic deficits, death	Arterial blood gas co-oximetry	Non-rebreather oxygen +/− Hyperbaric oxygen chamber therapy	Consider when multiple patients from same household have similar symptoms Hyperbaric oxygen therapy is indicated for neurologic or cardiovascular signs and above certain cutoffs
Space-occupying lesions	Progressively worsening headache History of malignancy Worse in morning or in head-down position	CT head MRI	Neurosurgical consultation ICP-lowering therapies Lesion-specific therapies	Emergent ICP-lowering therapies may include elevating head of bed, diuretics, and hyperventilation Lesion-specific therapies may include operative intervention, corticosteroids, and antimicrobial agents
Occult trauma	Signs of abuse or neglect Anticoagulation or coagulopathy	CT head	Neurosurgical consultation	Patients in at-risk populations (e.g., abuse) may not volunteer a history of trauma
Reversal cerebral vasoconstriction syndrome (RCVS)	Thunderclap headaches resolving within minutes or hours Multiple recurrent sudden, severe exacerbations are highly suggestive	CT or MR angiography	Supportive care, monitoring in neurosurgical ICU	Ischemic or hemorrhagic strokes can occur in 20% of patients Postpartum period is a risk factor (occurs in other patient populations as well)
Cerebellar infarction	Headache with dizziness Cerebellar signs Cranial nerve abnormalities	CT head MRI	Neurologic or neurosurgical consultation	Although CT head is insensitive for infarction, it is helpful initially to rule out hemorrhage and identify life-threatening edema and mass effect

Adapted directly from Raam and Tabatabai [10]

References

1. Doretti A, et al. Headaches in the emergency department—a survey of patients' characteristics, facts and needs. J Headache Pain. 2019;20(1):100. https://doi.org/10.1186/s10194-019-1053-5.
2. Goldstein J, Camargo C, Edlow J. Headache in United States emergency departments: demographics, work-up and frequency of pathological diagnoses. Cephalalgia. 2006;26(6):684–90. https://doi.org/10.1111/j.1468-2982.2006.01093.x.
3. Locker T, Mason S, Rigby A. Headache management—are we doing enough? An observational study of patients presenting with headache to the emergency department. Emerg Med J. 2004;21:327–32. https://doi.org/10.1136/emj.2003.012351.
4. The International Classification of Headache Disorders. Headache Classification Committee of the International Headache Society (IHS) The International Classification of Headache Disorders, 3rd edition. Cephalalgia. 2018;38(1):1–211. https://doi.org/10.1177/0333102417738202.
5. Ashina M. Migraine. N Engl J Med. 2020;383:1866–76. https://doi.org/10.1056/NEJMra1915327.
6. Charles A. Advances in the basic and clinical science of migraine Ann Neurol. 2009;65(5):491–8. https://doi.org/10.1002/ana.21691.
7. Ashina M, et al. Migraine and the trigeminovascular system—40 years and counting. Lancet Neurol. 2019;18:795–804. https://doi.org/10.1016/S1474-4422(19)30185-1.
8. Torres-Ferrus M, et al. From transformation to chronification of migraine: pathophysiological and clinical aspects. J Headache Pain. 2020;21(1):42. https://doi.org/10.1186/s10194-020-01111-8.
9. Munoz-Ceron J, et al. Headache at the emergency room: etiologies, diagnostic usefulness of the ICHD 3 criteria, red and green flags. PLoS One. 2019;14(1):e0208728. https://doi.org/10.1371/journal.pone.0208728.
10. Raam R, Tabatabai R. Headache in the emergency department: avoiding misdiagnosis of dangerous secondary causes, an update. Emerg Med Clin N Am. 2021;39(1):67–85. https://doi.org/10.1016/j.emc.2020.09.004.
11. Cutrer FM, Wippold FJ, Edlow JA. Evaluation of the adult with nontraumatic headache in the emergency department. In: Post TW, editor. UpToDate. Waltham: UpToDate Inc; 2019. http://www.uptodate.com.
12. Ramirez-Lassepas M, Espinosa CE, Cicero JJ, Johnston KL, Cipolle RJ, Barber DL. Predictors of intracranial pathologic findings in patients who seek emergency care because of headache. Arch Neurol. 1997;54(12):1506–9. https://doi.org/10.1001/archneur.1997.00550240058013.
13. Wolf SJ, et al. Clinical policy: critical issues in the evaluation and management of adult patients presenting to the emergency department with acute headache. Ann Emerg Med. 2019;74(4):e41–74. https://doi.org/10.1016/j.annemergmed.2019.07.009.
14. Pope J, Edlow J. Favorable response to analgesics does not predict a benign etiology of headache. Headache. 2008;48(6):944–50. https://doi.org/10.1111/j.1526-4610.2008.01127.x.
15. Pringsheim T, Becker W. Triptans for symptomatic treatment of migraine headache. BMJ. 2014;348:g2285. https://doi.org/10.1136/bmj.g2285.
16. Law S, Derry S, Moore RA. Sumatriptan plus naproxen for the treatment of acute migraine attacks in adults. Cochrane Database Syst Rev. 2016;4(4):CD008541. https://doi.org/10.1002/14651858.CD008541.pub3.
17. Lipton R, et al. Efficacy of rimegepant for the acute treatment of migraine based on triptan treatment experience: pooled results from three phase 3 randomized clinical trials. Cephalalgia. 2023;43(2):3310242211141686. https://doi.org/10.1177/03331024221141686.
18. Colman I, Friedman B, et al. Parenteral dexamethasone for acute severe migraine headache: meta-analysis of randomised controlled trials for preventing recurrence. BMJ. 2008;336(7657):1359.

19. Langer-Gould A, et al. The American Academy of Neurology's top five choosing wisely recommendations. Neurology. 2013;81(11):1004–11. https://doi.org/10.1212/WNL.0b013e31828aab14.
20. Weinman D, et al. Parenteral treatment of episodic tension-type headache: a systematic review. Headache. 2014;54(2):260–8. https://doi.org/10.1111/head.12287.
21. Cohen A, Burns B, Goadsby P. High-flow oxygen for treatment of cluster headache: a randomized trial. JAMA. 2009;302(22):2451–7. https://doi.org/10.1001/jama.2009.1855.
22. Law S, Derry S, Moore RA. Triptans for acute cluster headache. Cochrane Database Syst Rev. 2013;2013(7):CD008042. https://doi.org/10.1002/14651858.CD008042.pub3.
23. Miner JR, et al. Sumatriptan for the treatment of undifferentiated primary headaches in the ED. Am J Emerg Med. 2007;25(1):60. https://doi.org/10.1016/j.ajem.2006.06.004.
24. Torelli P, et al. Management of primary headaches in adult emergency departments; a literature review, the Parma ED experience and a therapy flow chart proposal. Neurol Sci. 2010;31(5):545–53. https://doi.org/10.1007/s10072-010-0337-y.

Eye Issues

2

Charles Hwang

2.1 Introduction

Ocular complaints are common in both the primary care office and emergency department settings and comprise approximately 2% of primary care patient visits [1, 2]. While most patients presenting with these symptoms will have a self-limiting etiology, vision-threatening and potentially rapidly progressing diagnoses are on the differential. The clinician must maintain a high degree of vigilance to properly rule out these conditions.

2.2 Differential Diagnosis

Condition	Acuity
Eyelid/periorbital conditions	
Blepharitis	Routine
Chalazion	Routine
Dacryoadenitis	Routine
Dacryocystitis	Routine
Hordeolum (stye)	Routine
Orbital cellulitis	Emergent
Preseptal (periorbital) cellulitis	Routine
Xanthelasma	Routine
Red/painful eye	
Traumatic	
Chemical burns	Urgent vs. emergent
Corneal abrasions	Routine
Corneal foreign bodies	Situationally dependent

C. Hwang (✉)
Department of Emergency Medicine, University of Florida College of Medicine
Gainesville, FL, USA
e-mail: hwang.c@ufl.edu

B. K. Desai et al. (eds.), *Primary Care for Emergency Physicians*,
https://doi.org/10.1007/978-3-031-64676-8_2

Condition	Acuity
Globe rupture	Emergent
Hyphema	Urgent
Subconjunctival hemorrhage	Routine
Atraumatic	
Acute angle-closure glaucoma	Emergent
Conjunctivitis (bacterial, viral, allergic)	Routine
Corneal ulcer	Urgent
Dry eye (keratoconjunctivitis sicca)	Routine
Endophthalmitis	Emergent
Episcleritis	Urgent
Hypopyon	Emergent
Iritis (anterior uveitis)	Urgent
Keratitis	Emergent
Pterygium	Routine
Scleritis	Urgent
Loss of vision	
Painful	
Giant cell arteritis (temporal arteritis)	Urgent
Optic neuritis	Urgent
Painless	
Central retinal artery occlusion (CRAO)	Emergent
Retinal detachment	Emergent

2.3 History

A full ophthalmologic history should be obtained in all patients with ocular/periorbital complaints. Like other organ systems, it is important to clarify history elements with the patient, with close attention to specific anatomic structures involved (e.g., eye vs. eyelid vs. periorbital structures) and symptoms (e.g., does "something in the eye" refer to something the patient sees when they visualize the eye or something they notice in their vision? Is diplopia monocular or binocular? Does the visual disturbance only occur with near or distance reading?). It is important to distinguish if the symptoms involve one or both eyes. Systemic diseases and age-related processes typically affect both eyes, although the presentation and/or progression may affect one eye more significantly. In contrast, infectious or vascular processes typically have unilateral involvement, particularly in the early stages [3]. Key components of the general medical history include the use of any anticoagulants and the presence of systemic disease with potential ocular manifestations, such as sarcoidosis, human immunodeficiency virus (HIV), tuberculosis (TB), and rheumatoid arthritis.

A history of sudden vision loss or decrease should prompt emergent specialist consultation. A description of a curtain or veil being pulled across the visual field, as well as new-onset or worsening floaters, suggests a retinal detachment. Sudden visual loss, particularly in a patient with atrial fibrillation or other cerebrovascular accident risk factors, suggests a central retinal artery occlusion. Vitreous hemorrhage and central retinal vein occlusion may also result in abrupt, painless vision loss.

Other important historical features to elicit include:

Diplopia (monocular vs. binocular, near vs. distance, certain directions of gaze)
Discharge
  Amount
  Consistency
  Worsening in AM
Discomfort
  Aggravation or alleviation of symptoms with blinking
  Foreign body sensation
  Itching
Exposures
  Chemical
    *Red flag: Alkali and other caustic exposures
  Ultraviolet light (including skiing/high altitudes, welding)
Genitourinary symptoms: may suggest chlamydial or gonorrheal disease
Location (eye vs. eyelid vs. periorbital structures)
Photophobia
Trauma
Upper respiratory infection symptoms
Vision
Vomiting
  *Red flag: Highly suspicious for angle-closure glaucoma if associated with visual disturbance and/or red eye

2.4 Physical Exam

Visual acuity is the vital sign of the eye and should be assessed in any patient presenting with an ocular complaint. The visual acuity should be measured separately for each eye. If the patient's prescribed glasses are not at bedside, visual acuity measured through a pinhole will suffice [2]. An orderly progression through the physical examination of the periorbital region and the eye can then ensue as outlined below.

Pitfall: Following a traumatic injury, the integrity of the globe must immediately be assessed. The presence of pupillary irregularity (particularly a teardrop-shaped pupil), a corneal or scleral laceration, a positive Seidel's test, or a flat anterior chamber should prompt cessation of any further manipulation of the globe and immediate ophthalmology consultation.

2.4.1 Periorbital Exam

Discharge
  *Red flag: Copious purulent discharge in patients with risk factors for sexually transmitted diseases (gonorrheal conjunctivitis)
Edema

Erythema
Lid eversion
*Red flag: In patients with foreign body sensation or corneal abrasion with concern for retained foreign body, lid eversion should be performed to evaluate for foreign body
Papular lesions (e.g., hordeolum, chalazion)
Proptosis
*Red flag: Proptosis is associated with retrobulbar mass effect (e.g., hemorrhage in the setting of trauma, orbital cellulitis), cavernous sinus thrombosis, and malignancy
Vesicular rash (herpes zoster virus [HZV])
*Red flag: Hutchinson's sign, a vesicular lesion on the tip of the nose, is highly associated with herpes zoster ophthalmicus (HZO)

2.4.2 Extraocular Movements

*Red flag: Restriction of movement is associated with retrobulbar mass effect (e.g., orbital cellulitis or retrobulbar hemorrhage), traumatic entrapment, or cranial nerve palsies

2.4.3 Conjunctival and Sclera Evaluation

Chemosis
Conjunctival injection (presence or absence of limbal injection)
Foreign bodies
Laceration (*Red flag for globe rupture)
Scleral injection
Subconjunctival hemorrhage

2.4.4 Pupil Exam

Photophobia
Reactivity: Assess for an afferent pupillary defect (Marcus Gunn Pupil). An afferent pupillary defect is present if the affected eye dilates in response to direct light and constricts in response to consensual light. Conditions affecting the retina, optic nerve, optic chiasm, and optic tract may result in this finding [4].
The pupil is fixed and mid-dilated in cases of acute angle-closure glaucoma.
Shape
*Red flag: An irregularly shaped pupil, particularly a teardrop shape, strongly suggests globe rupture
Size

Subtle (<1 mm discrepancy) anisocoria is physiologic in approximately 20% of patients but may also result from third nerve palsy due to uncal herniation, Horner's syndrome, medications, and direct trauma [2].

2.4.5 Corneal Examination

Fluorescein uptake
 Abrasions
 Dendritic lesions
  *Red flag for herpes simplex virus (HSV) ophthalmicus
 Seidel's sign (dye streaming from injury site)
  *Red flag for globe rupture
 Ulcer
Foreign bodies
Opacities

2.4.6 Intraocular Pressure

Normal 10–20 mmHg

*Red flag: Increased intraocular pressure suggests acute angle-closure glaucoma in the appropriate clinical scenario

Pitfall: Do not attempt to measure intraocular pressure if there is any concern for globe rupture

Pitfall: Falsely elevated pressure may result if any pressure is placed on globe by examiner during measurement

2.4.7 Slit Lamp Examination

Cell and flare (presence of white blood cells and protein in anterior chamber) suggest iritis

Depth of anterior chamber

Presence of red blood cells (hyphema) or white blood cells (hypopyon) in the anterior chamber

2.4.8 Funduscopic Exam

Papilledema: *Red flag

Retinal detachment: *Red flag

Retinal hemorrhage: *Red flag

Retinal pallor: *Red flag for central retinal artery occlusion (particularly if associated with "cherry red spot")

Pitfall: In general, a dilated exam should only be performed by an ophthalmologist. Do not dilate if there is any concern for acute angle-closure glaucoma

2.5 Specific Conditions and Their Management

2.5.1 Eyelid/Periorbital Conditions

2.5.1.1 Blepharitis

Acute or chronic inflammation of the hair follicles and meibomian glands at the lid margin, commonly associated with staphylococcal infection, is termed blepharitis. It is characterized by edema, erythema, pruritus, "pink eyes," excessive tearing and discharge, and crusting/matting of the eyelashes and lid margin. Conjunctival injection may be present. Symptoms are typically most severe in the morning. Application of warm compresses and gentle cleaning with baby shampoo are typically effective. In refractory cases, the use of topical antibiotics can be considered [5–8].

2.5.1.2 Hordeolum and Chalazion

A hordeolum (commonly referred to as a stye) is a painful and erythematous eyelid mass resulting from acute bacterial infection. An external hordeolum is a lesion originating from the glands of Zeis or Moll. An internal hordeolum is caused by meibomian gland inflammation. *Staphylococcus aureus* is the most commonly identified pathogen. In most cases, hordeola are self-limited, and warm compresses applied several times daily are first-line therapy. Lid hygiene after warm compresses can facilitate drainage. Topical bacitracin can also be considered. If persistent despite these measures, patients may be referred to an ophthalmologist for incision and drainage [9, 10].

Obstruction of a meibomian gland can result in formation of a chronic inflammatory lesion at the lid border termed a chalazion. The skin itself is typically normal; however, lid edema and/or a discrete nodular lesion may be noted. The presence of pain should suggest an alternative diagnosis. Warm compresses can be applied, but the lesions are typically self-limited. Antibiotics are not indicated. If large and persistent, incision and drainage by an ophthalmologist can be considered [6, 9].

2.5.1.3 Dacryoadenitis and Dacryocystitis

Infection of the lacrimal glands is termed dacryoadenitis, while infection of the lacrimal sac is termed dacryocystitis. Patients with dacryoadenitis typically present with abrupt onset eyelid edema, particularly near the upper lid margin. Dacryocystitis is typically preceded by an upper respiratory infection with development of erythema and edema just inferior to the medial canthus occurring several days later. Fever is typically present. With either condition, patients can appear quite ill.

A variety of pathogens, both viral and bacterial, can be responsible for either. *S. aureus* is the most common bacterial etiology in dacryoadenitis. In neonates, *Streptococcus pneumoniae* is the predominant etiology, and *S. aureus* and *Staphylococcus epidermidis* are more common in older children and adults. Prompt treatment of dacryoadenitis and dacryocystitis with systemic antibiotics is crucial to prevent secondary complications. Therapy of dacryoadenitis includes parenteral antibiotics with anti-staphylococcal coverage. Methicillin-resistant *S. aureus* (MRSA) coverage should be added as appropriate based on local susceptibility patterns. Patients with dacryocystitis typically require parenteral antibiotics. Infants, in particular, require admission to the hospital [9, 11].

2.5.1.4 Preseptal (Periorbital) and Orbital Cellulitis

Cellulitis affecting the area surrounding the eye is divided into preseptal (periorbital) or orbital cellulitis depending on the presence of infection posterior to the orbital septum. Orbital cellulitis is acutely life- and sight-threatening; therefore, differentiating the two entities is crucial. Some clinicians use the term "periorbital cellulitis" and "preseptal cellulitis" interchangeably; however, because of the clinical implications and morbidity associated with orbital cellulitis, we prefer the term "preseptal cellulitis" over "periorbital cellulitis" to obviate any confusion between the distinct disease entities.

Preseptal cellulitis is typically more indolent in development and often preceded by minor skin trauma or a cutaneous facial infection such as a hordeolum. Orbital cellulitis is much more commonly abrupt in onset and the result of extension of sinusitis. Erythema, edema, and warmth surrounding the affected eye, as well as fever, may be present in both entities. The presence of visual changes, proptosis, and restriction of extraocular movement, as well as pain associated with such movement, suggest orbital cellulitis and/or abscess formation. If orbital cellulitis is suspected, patients should be emergently evaluated with CT or MRI to establish the presence or absence of inflammatory changes posterior to the orbital septum.

In a well-appearing patient with preseptal cellulitis, treatment with an oral antibiotic regimen active against both MRSA and *S. pneumoniae* and *Haemophilus influenzae* is appropriate [6]. Amoxicillin/clavulanate along with sulfamethoxazole/trimethoprim or clindamycin is an appropriate regimen. Patients who do not experience improvement in symptoms within 24 h should be reassessed for evidence of orbital cellulitis. Patients with orbital cellulitis require hospital admission, broad-spectrum parenteral antibiotics, and ophthalmology consultation.

2.5.2 Intrinsic Orbit Conditions: *Traumatic Injuries*

2.5.2.1 Globe Rupture

Globe rupture involves compromise in the integrity of the cornea and/or sclera [12]. A globe rupture should be suspected after any high-impact blunt or penetrating injury to the orbit or periorbital region. Other traumatic injuries may coexist depending on the mechanism of injury. Signs and symptoms of globe rupture include eye pain, decreased visual acuity, hyphema, and an irregular or asymmetric pupil. The depth of the anterior chamber may be decreased. A fluorescein stain should be performed to evaluate for Seidel's sign; a positive test would show dilution of the fluorescent dye near the defect under cobalt blue examination and suggests full-thickness corneal or scleral injury. It is important to note that globe rupture may be occult, and a low threshold for further evaluation and consultation should be maintained if the diagnosis is suspected despite lack of the cardinal findings noted above.

CT of the orbits is the typical next study in such cases. MRI is contraindicated if there is any concern for a metallic foreign body. Management includes emergent ophthalmology consultation, broad-spectrum parenteral antibiotics (e.g., vancomycin and a fourth-generation cephalosporin), and placement of an eye shield. No further manipulation of the globe should occur unless undertaken by an ophthalmologist. Provide adequate analgesia and update tetanus immunization status as appropriate. Patients should remain NPO. Elevate the head of the patient's bed and treat any nausea or vomiting to protect against elevation of intraocular pressure.

2.5.2.2 Hyphema

Blood in the anterior chamber following a traumatic injury is an indication for urgent ophthalmology evaluation. In the interim, patients should be evaluated for evidence of any other traumatic injuries. If no contraindication exists, patients should be advised to sit upright to minimize the staining of the cornea. Pain control should be administered (avoid topical agents if globe rupture is suspected). Due to rebleeding risk, NSAIDs and aspirin are contraindicated. Treat nausea and limit potential pupillary accommodation/constriction, which can result in further bleeding, by dimming/reducing ambient light. An eye shield can be utilized.

2.5.2.3 Subconjunctival Hemorrhage

While the characteristic appearance of extravasated blood associated with a subconjunctival hemorrhage is often alarming to patients, the condition is typically benign. Patients may notice this finding after a direct traumatic injury, coughing, vomiting, or Valsalva. Alternatively, the onset can be spontaneous. Subconjunctival hemorrhage is painless, and the presence of pain should prompt a search for an alternative/coexisting diagnosis, particularly in the setting of trauma. Evaluate for a corneal abrasion in these patients, and consider the possibility of an open globe injury. If the patient is anticoagulated, consider assessment of coagulation parameters. Reassurance of patients is indicated, as is counseling that up to 2–3 weeks may be needed for full resorption of the blood [5].

2.5.2.4 Corneal Abrasions

Intense pain and photophobia are the most common presenting complaints among patients presenting with corneal abrasions. A history of eye trauma immediately preceding the onset of symptoms is often apparent. It is crucial to evaluate for more sinister injuries, particularly an occult open globe or hyphema, in the setting of a significant traumatic mechanism. Unfortunately, the physical exam, including measurement of visual acuity, is often limited by the patient's presenting symptoms. If there is no evidence of an open globe, a dose of topical anesthetic (e.g., proparacaine 0.5%) should be administered and will provide near immediate relief. Despite their efficacy, continued use of these agents is contraindicated due to concern for epithelial toxicity [13]. Subsequent fluorescein instillation will allow for enhancement of the abrasion under a Wood's lamp or the cobalt blue filter of an ophthalmoscope or slit lamp. The presence or absence of a Seidel's sign should be assessed concurrently. Eversion of the upper eyelid to evaluate for a retained foreign body is warranted.

Adequate analgesia is important for all patients. Most small abrasions will heal completely within 24 h at which time patients should be pain-free. In the interim, oral NSAIDs and/or opiate analgesia can be prescribed. Topical NSAIDs are also appropriate, although their cost can be significant. There is no evidence that patching of abrasions, especially small lesions, leads to improvement in rate of healing or pain control [14]. Contact lens wearers should never be patched. Larger abrasions require a longer course of oral analgesia. An ophthalmologist may consider the use of a cycloplegic agent in such cases.

Appropriate antibiotic coverage should be administered. In abrasions associated with contact lens use, patients should receive coverage for *Pseudomonas aeruginosa* (e.g., moxifloxacin, one to two drops three times daily for 7 days). Appropriate coverage for others includes polymyxin-trimethoprim or erythromycin ointment (one drop or 0.5 inch, respectively, four times daily for 3–5 days).

Patients with a hypopyon (WBCs in the anterior chamber), hyphema, or corneal ulceration should be evaluated by an ophthalmologist emergently. Urgent referral is warranted for corneal abrasions without healing after 3–4 days, patients with a significant decrease in visual acuity, large abrasions (>one quarter of the diameter of the cornea), and those with purulent discharge.

2.5.2.5 Corneal Foreign Body

Corneal foreign bodies characteristically present with severe eye irritation worsened with blinking. Conjunctival injection, photophobia, and increased lacrimation are typically also present. Evaluate for a ruptured globe prior to any attempt at foreign body removal. Following application of topical anesthetic, attempts at foreign body removal can be made with irrigation or use of a moistened cotton swab. If unsuccessful, a clinician with experience in corneal foreign body removal with a 25-gauge needle or eye spud under magnification can make an additional attempt. Metallic foreign bodies present for more than several hours can result in formation of a rust ring. If such a ring is noted following foreign body removal, the patient should be referred to an ophthalmologist within the next several days. There is no need for emergent rust ring removal provided prompt ophthalmology follow-up is available. Urgent ophthalmology consultation is indicated for patients with foreign bodies which cannot be easily removed. All patients should be referred to ophthalmology on an outpatient basis to evaluate for delayed presentation of infection. Provide oral analgesia and topical antibiotics as would be given for a patient with a corneal abrasion [7, 15].

2.5.2.6 Chemical Burns

Any exposure of the globe to caustic material is a true ophthalmic emergency. Alkali exposures are particularly dangerous as they result in liquefactive necrosis, permitting deeper progression of damage, compared to the coagulative necrosis caused by acidic substances. The initial treatment for all chemical burns is copious irrigation with normal saline, preferably via a Morgan lens. Topical anesthesia (e.g., proparacaine) can be administered to reduce pain and irritation and facilitate irrigation. Do not delay irrigation to obtain visual acuity or other testing. Following 30 min of irrigation, ocular pH should be checked using litmus paper. Continue irrigation until the eye has maintained a pH of 7.0 for at least 30 min. It is prudent to evert the eyelid to evaluate for the possibility of retained or crystallized particulate matter, which may result in persistent difficulties in achieving a neutral pH. Immediate ophthalmology consultation is indicated in all cases of caustic exposure [7, 16].

2.5.3 Intrinsic Orbit Conditions: *Atraumatic Conditions*

2.5.3.1 Acute Angle-Closure Glaucoma

An abrupt increase in intraocular pressure can result from impaired drainage of aqueous humor in anatomically predisposed individuals (typically patients with hyperopia). Typical precipitants include dim lighting and medications with the side effect of pupillary dilatation (e.g., anticholinergics). This pressure increase can be acutely sight-threatening and demands emergent reversal. Symptoms include blurred vision, visualization of colored halos near lights, nausea, vomiting, frontal headache, and severe eye pain. On physical exam, conjunctival injection, a fixed mid-dilated pupil, and a hazy cornea may be appreciated. If available, tonometry should be conducted by the clinician; if unavailable, emergent referral to an ophthalmologist is indicated. In acute angle-closure glaucoma, intraocular pressure is typically >30 mmHg. Pending ophthalmologic evaluation, systemic acetazolamide can be given as well as consideration of topical timolol, apraclonidine, and/or pilocarpine. Laser peripheral iridotomy is the typical definitive treatment [16].

2.5.3.2 Conjunctivitis

Viral conjunctivitis is the most common cause of a red eye [17], although bacterial infection and allergic mechanisms are also commonly responsible. Discerning the etiology responsible for a specific case of conjunctivitis can be difficult. Inflammation of the conjunctiva almost universally results in redness and discharge of the affected eye(s), as well as matting of the eyelids upon awakening, regardless of etiology. Itching of the eyes in the setting of other conjunctivitis symptoms is a distinguishing factor implicating an allergic etiology. Bacterial infection is more common in children than adults. Concomitant or preceding upper respiratory infection symptoms suggest adenoviral conjunctivitis. Clinicians should be vigilant in performing a systematic and detailed physical exam in patients with conjunctivitis, with special attention to fluorescein staining to rule out more serious pathology which patients and/or parents will typically ascribe to "pink eye."

Viral conjunctivitis is most commonly caused by one of many strains of adenovirus, although HSV can cause particularly severe disease as discussed below. Adenoviral conjunctivitis is highly contagious, potentially transmissible up to 2 weeks following onset of symptoms. Strict hand hygiene is therefore indicated. Topical antibiotics are not necessary, as bacterial superinfection is rare and patients can be expected to have spontaneous resolution of symptoms generally within several days, with occasional persistence up to 2 weeks.

The most common bacterial etiology is *S. aureus* in older children and adults, while *H. influenzae, S. pneumoniae*, and *Moraxella catarrhalis* predominate in young children [18]. Preferred antibacterial agents for nonusers of contact lenses are erythromycin ointment (0.5 inches applied four times daily) or polymyxin-trimethoprim (one to two drops applied four times daily). A 5–7-day course is typically prescribed. Topical aminoglycosides are generally avoided due to their inherent toxicity to the corneal epithelium and tendency to cause further irritation with prolonged use. The presence of a concomitant acute otitis media, particularly in children, implies *H. influenzae* infection. Affected patients should also be treated with systemic antibiotics with activity against this pathogen (e.g., amoxicillin/clavulanate).

P. aeruginosa is a common pathogen in contact lens wearers. Such patients are also at high risk of corneal ulceration and keratitis, and a thorough evaluation for these conditions is indicated, as their presence necessitates prompt ophthalmology consultation. In the absence of these findings, management in contact lens users typically employs topical fluoroquinolones. Patients should be advised to discard the lenses they were using just prior to symptom development and to avoid use of any lens until cleared to do so by an ophthalmologist. If there is no improvement in symptoms after 12–24 h of treatment, urgent ophthalmology referral is indicated.

Chlamydial conjunctivitis should be suspected in at-risk patients refractory to standard bacterial conjunctivitis treatment. Infection occurs through contact either directly from the genitalia or via the hands. Symptoms of coexisting genital tract disease are variably present. Systemic therapy (azithromycin 1 g PO X 1 or doxycycline 100 mg PO bid X 7 days) to clear the genital infection as well as topical therapy (e.g., erythromycin) should be administered. Sexual contacts should also be tested and treated [5, 17].

Hyperacute bacterial conjunctivitis, typically associated with *Neisseria gonorrhoeae*, is often heralded by a very abrupt onset of copious discharge from the affected eye(s) after introduction of the pathogen (≤12 h). Spread is similar to that noted with chlamydial disease. Urethritis symptoms are often present. Cultures should be obtained, and topical antibiotics (e.g., erythromycin) as well as systemic ceftriaxone (1 g IM) should be administered. Due to the high risk of complications including corneal perforation and blindness, immediate ophthalmology consultation is warranted [17].

Children born in US hospitals typically receive erythromycin ointment immediately after birth to reduce the likelihood of gonococcal ophthalmia neonatorum. This condition most commonly presents during the first week of life with the onset of copious purulent eye discharge and conjunctival injection. Patients may present overtly septic due to disseminated infection. Systemic ceftriaxone should be administered, and patients should be admitted to the hospital with emergent ophthalmology consultation. Chlamydial conjunctivitis typically presents somewhat later (days 5–14) than conjunctivitis secondary to gonorrhea. Pneumonia is commonly associated. Oral and topical erythromycin should be administered, and ophthalmology should be urgently consulted. Untreated, corneal scarring can result [19].

Allergic conjunctivitis can be caused by environmental allergens such as pollen, as well as through contact with irritating topical medications. In addition to the general supportive care recommendations for all patients with conjunctivitis, topical and/or systemic antihistamines and a topical vasoconstrictor can be utilized. However, identification and avoidance of possible triggers are absolutely indicated.

2.5.3.3 Corneal Ulcer

A deep infection of the cornea secondary to epithelial disruption due to direct bacterial invasion, trauma, or sloughing of cells due to desiccation (e.g., with incomplete lid closure due to Bell's palsy) is termed a corneal ulcer. Soft contact lens wearers are at particularly high risk. Pain, photophobia, and foreign body sensation are typical symptoms. An area of white discoloration of the cornea is often appreciated; the lesion will enhance with fluorescein under a Wood's lamp. *P. aeruginosa* is of particular concern in contact lens wearers, while *S. pneumoniae* and *S. aureus* are typical culprits in other patients. Urgent ophthalmology consultation is indicated. A topical fluoroquinolone, with very frequent application, is typically prescribed following culture of the lesion [7, 19].

2.5.3.4 Endophthalmitis

Endophthalmitis refers to a bacterial or fungal infection within the eye, including involvement of the aqueous and/or vitreous humors. Most cases of endophthalmitis result from direct inoculation by exogenous sources, such as trauma, injection, surgery, or direct spread (e.g., keratitis). The remaining cases are the result of hematogenous spread [12].

Patients with endophthalmitis due to recent ocular surgery usually manifest symptoms within a week of surgery. Signs and symptoms may include rapid progression of decreased vision, eye pain, conjunctival injection or chemosis, eye discharge, and hypopyon. The clinical outcome depends on the causative organism and the timeliness of definitive therapy; therefore, emergent ophthalmologic evaluation is essential.

2.5.3.5 Episcleritis and Scleritis

Differentiating episcleritis from scleritis is key, as the former is a generally benign condition, while the latter (which can also affect deeper structures of the globe) is potentially sight-threatening. Features of episcleritis include onset of excessive lacrimation, irritation, and eye redness which typically only affect a segment of the globe. This stands in contrast to the more diffuse redness associated with conjunctivitis. Scleritis is typically associated with severe pain, an important distinguishing feature from the "grittiness" or mild irritation that patients with episcleritis may report. Scleritis is often associated with systemic disease, specifically rheumatoid arthritis and Wegener's granulomatosis. If scleritis is suspected, urgent referral to ophthalmology is warranted. Treatment typically consists of systemic NSAIDs, glucocorticoids, or other immunosuppressants [20]. Although episcleritis is typically self-limited, topical lubricants, with or without topical NSAIDs, are often employed for symptomatic relief.

2.5.3.6 Keratitis

Inflammation of the cornea is termed keratitis. Patients commonly present with severe pain, photophobia, and eye redness. Herpes simplex virus (typically reactivation rather than primary infection) is the most common cause; however, other viruses, bacteria, UV radiation, and incomplete closure of the eyelid (e.g., with Bell's palsy) are also responsible. Contact lens wearers are at increased risk due to *P. aeruginosa*. Herpes simplex infection involving the cornea is associated with ulceration and a characteristic dendritic pattern noted on fluorescein staining. Typical herpetic lesions may be present on the conjunctiva and eyelids. Treatment includes topical antivirals (e.g., trifluridine 1% nine times daily). Patients with bacterial or viral keratitis should be seen by an ophthalmologist urgently on a same-day basis [7, 19].

Ultraviolet keratitis is associated with welding, skiing, and high-altitude exposure. Symptom onset is typically within 6–12 h of the insult. Avoidance of triggers and use of eye protection should be advised. Oral analgesia should be prescribed, and the patient should be referred for outpatient ophthalmology follow-up.

Pitfalls: Only ophthalmologists should prescribe topical ophthalmic steroids. In the case of herpes simplex virus infection, topical steroid use can result in deeper involvement of eye structures and permanent visual impairment.

Beware of the possibility of topical anesthetic abuse among patients with frequent exposure to insults which result in UV keratitis. Never prescribe topical anesthetic drops given the potential for corneal epithelial toxicity.

2.5.3.7 Iritis (Anterior Uveitis)

Iritis is commonly associated with infectious and systemic diseases such as herpes viruses, tuberculosis, syphilis, spondyloarthritides, and sarcoidosis. Traumatic injuries may also be causative. The pupil is typically constricted and sluggishly reactive. Symptoms include pain, blurred vision, and conjunctival injection. Eye discharge is typically scant if present. A key exam finding is consensual photophobia (pain when light is exposed to the unaffected eye due to constriction of the iris). On slit lamp examination, a "cell and flare" pattern due to the presence of white blood cells and proteinaceous material in the anterior chamber may be noted. In more severe infection, white blood cells may settle in the anterior chamber resulting in accumulation of a hypopyon. Sequelae of the diagnosis include glaucoma and cataract formation. Urgent ophthalmology consultation is warranted.

2.5.3.8 Herpes Zoster Ophthalmicus

Herpes zoster ophthalmicus refers to reactivation of latent varicella zoster virus in the ophthalmic division of cranial nerve V. Patients often experience a prodrome of fatigue, as well as pain affecting the dermatome in the days prior to rash onset. Hutchinson's sign, the presence of vesicles on the tip of the nose, is associated with a higher likelihood of ocular involvement. Ocular manifestations can include blepharitis, conjunctivitis, keratitis, scleritis, iritis, retinitis, and optic neuritis. Management includes urgent ophthalmology consultation if there is any evidence of ocular involvement and administration of systemic antivirals (e.g., acyclovir 800 mg PO five times daily for 7–10 days). Antivirals are most efficacious when started within 72 h of onset of rash. Adequate analgesia should also be administered. Hospitalization and IV antivirals should be considered for the immunocompromised and those with severe disease (e.g., retinitis) [21].

2.5.3.9 Pterygium

A wedge-shaped proliferation of conjunctival tissue which extends onto the cornea is termed a pterygium. The pathogenesis is unclear; however, excessive exposure to UV radiation is a known risk factor. The symptoms are typically slowly progressive and the lesion itself is painless. However, patients may present due to cosmetic concerns, eye irritation, and potentially vision loss due to covering of the visual axis or induced astigmatism. Patients with eye irritation should be counseled to use eye lubrication. In the event of visual disturbance, non-emergent ophthalmological referral is appropriate for consideration of removal [17].

2.5.4 Loss of Vision: *Painful*

2.5.4.1 Giant Cell Arteritis (Temporal Arteritis)

Giant cell arteritis (GCA, temporal arteritis) is a systemic vasculitis that principally affects individuals older than 50 years of age. Because GCA is a systemic vasculitis, the signs and symptoms may be widespread, diffuse, nonspecific, and variable over time; cranial involvement, however, results in the feared complication of vision loss (up to 15–25%) if left untreated [12]. Therefore, a high index of suspicion must be maintained.

The systemic symptoms present subacutely and may include constitutional symptoms of low-grade fever, malaise, fatigue, weight loss, a headache that is new in character, and jaw claudication. Ocular complaints may include transient monocular vision loss (e.g., visual field defect or amaurosis fugax—a temporary curtain over the field of vision). The patient may exhibit temporal tenderness.

For the diagnosis of GCA, a patient must have three out of the five American College of Rheumatology diagnostic criteria: age ≥50 years, new-onset headache, temporal artery abnormality (tenderness to palpation, decreased pulsation), elevated erythrocyte sedimentation rate (ESR) ≥50 mm/h, or abnormal temporal artery biopsy [22]. If the suspicion for GCA is high, treatment should not be delayed while awaiting a temporal artery biopsy. Rather, a patient should be referred to the emergency department for rheumatology and ophthalmology evaluation. The treatment of GCA is oral or parenteral steroids administered in conjunction with expert consultation.

2.5.4.2 Optic Neuritis

Optic neuritis is caused by the inflammatory demyelination of the optic nerve. It is often associated with multiple sclerosis but can also be associated with infectious, inflammatory, or autoimmune disorders. It typically affects younger individuals. Symptoms are usually monocular, and patients may experience subacute (hours to several days) vision loss, ocular pain especially with movement of the eye, a relative afferent pupillary defect, a visual field defect, and abnormal color vision.

The diagnosis of optic neuritis is clinical based on the above signs and symptoms. Patients should be urgently referred to an ophthalmologist for a dilated fundoscopic exam and a neurologist and magnetic resonance imaging (MRI) to evaluate for demyelinating lesions. The treatment for optic neuritis includes parenteral and oral steroids [12].

2.5.5 Loss of Vision: *Painless*

2.5.5.1 Central Retinal Artery Occlusion (CRAO)

Central retinal artery occlusion (CRAO) is acute painless vision loss due to retinal ischemia. It shares similar etiologies with cerebrovascular disease, such as carotid atherosclerosis and cardioembolic disease, although inflammatory conditions can contribute as well. Because CRAO causes irreversible ischemic damage to the retina in as little as 90 min [16, 23], it is considered an "ocular stroke" and is a medical and ophthalmologic emergency [12].

Symptoms include sudden, profound, monocular, painless vision loss. If a distal smaller artery is involved, the monocular vision loss may be partial. The patient may report a history of similar but transient episodes in the recent past. Signs include a relative afferent pupillary defect. Fundoscopic exam demonstrates a pale retina due to retinal ischemia and a "cherry red" macula. A "box-car" appearance may be visualized in the retinal vessels due to sluggish blood flow.

CRAO has a poor prognosis for vision. Efforts should be undertaken immediately to restore perfusion, although there are no proven therapies for CRAO, and these efforts are usually ineffective. Anecdotally, treatment options include intra-arterial thrombolysis, ocular massage to dislodge clot burden, reduction of intraocular pressure by eyedrops or anterior chamber paracentesis, vasodilatory medications, and inhalation of carbogen (95% O_2 and 5% CO_2). Ultimately, risk factor modification to prevent future cerebrovascular events is essential [12, 24].

2.5.5.2 Retinal Detachment

Retinal detachment (RD) is defined as the separation of the neurosensory layer of the retina from its underlying pigment epithelium. Left untreated, RD can result in permanent vision loss. Symptoms of RD include bright flashes of light in the peripheral vision, a sudden increase in the number of floaters, decreased visual acuity, or a dark curtain or shadow moving from the periphery to the central vision. Risk factors include increased age, high myopia, trauma, lattice degeneration, personal or family history of RD, diabetes, and connective tissue disorders [12].

Posterior vitreous detachment (PVD) presents similarly with flashers and floaters. PVD is an age-related process in which the vitreous humor degenerates and retracts from the retina and commonly occurs after the age of 40. If the PVD does not separate cleanly and completely from the retina, the PVD can provide traction on the retina, resulting in an RD. Therefore, any patient presenting with signs or symptoms concerning for PVD or RD should be evaluated by an ophthalmologist immediately.

References

1. Shields T, Sloane PD. A comparison of eye problems in primary care and ophthalmology practices. Fam Med. 1991;23:544–6.
2. Robinett DA, Kahn JH. The physical examination of the eye. Emerg Med Clin N Am. 2008;26:1–16. https://doi.org/10.1016/j.emc.2007.11.007.
3. Bradford CA, Melson AT. Ocular complaints, disease, and emergencies in the general medical setting. Med Clin N Am. 2021;105:409–23. https://doi.org/10.1016/j.mcna.2021.02.002.
4. Duong DK, Leo MM, Mitchell EL. Neuro-ophthalmology. Emerg Med Clin N Am. 2008;26:137–80. https://doi.org/10.1016/j.emc.2007.11.004.
5. Cronau H, Kankanala RR, Mauger T. Diagnosis and management of red eye in primary care. Am Fam Physician. 2010;81:137–44.
6. Carlisle RT, Digiovanni J. Differential diagnosis of the swollen red eyelid. Am Fam Physician. 2015;92:106–12.
7. Wirbelauer C. Management of the red eye for the primary care physician. Am J Med. 2006;119:302–6. https://doi.org/10.1016/j.amjmed.2005.07.065.
8. Duncan K, Jeng BH. Medical management of blepharitis. Curr Opin Ophthalmol. 2015;26:289–94. https://doi.org/10.1097/ICU.0000000000000164.
9. Wald ER. Periorbital and orbital infections. Infect Dis Clin N Am. 2007;21:393–408. https://doi.org/10.1016/j.idc.2007.03.008.
10. Lindsley K, Nichols JJ, Dickersin K. Non-surgical interventions for acute internal hordeolum. Cochrane Database Syst Rev. 2017;1:CD007742. https://doi.org/10.1002/14651858.CD007742.pub4.
11. Sethuraman U, Kamat D. The red eye: evaluation and management. Clin Pediatr. 2009;48:588–600. https://doi.org/10.1177/0009922809333094.
12. Shah SM, Khanna CL. Ophthalmic emergencies for the clinician. Mayo Clin Proc. 2020;95:1050–8. https://doi.org/10.1016/j.mayocp.2020.03.018.
13. Yagci A, Bozkurt B, Egrilmez S, Palamar M, Ozturk BT, Pekel H. Topical anesthetic abuse keratopathy: a commonly overlooked health care problem. Cornea. 2011;30:571–5. https://doi.org/10.1097/ICO.0b013e3182000af9.
14. Turner A, Rabiu M. Patching for corneal abrasion. In: Turner A, editor. Cochrane database of systematic reviews. Chichester: Wiley; 2006. https://doi.org/10.1002/14651858.CD004764.pub2.
15. Wipperman JL, Dorsch JN. Evaluation and management of corneal abrasions. Am Fam Physician. 2013;87:114–20.
16. Pokhrel PK, Loftus SA. Ocular emergencies. Am Fam Physician. 2007;76:829–36.
17. Leibowitz HM. The red eye. N Engl J Med. 2000;343:345–51. https://doi.org/10.1056/NEJM200008033430507.

18. Høvding G. Acute bacterial conjunctivitis. Acta Ophthalmol. 2008;86:5–17. https://doi.org/10.1111/j.1600-0420.2007.01006.x.
19. Deibel JP, Cowling K. Ocular inflammation and infection. Emerg Med Clin N Am. 2013;31:387–97. https://doi.org/10.1016/j.emc.2013.01.006.
20. Okhravi N, Odufuwa B, McCluskey P, Lightman S. Scleritis. Surv Ophthalmol. 2005;50:351–63. https://doi.org/10.1016/j.survophthal.2005.04.001.
21. Shaikh S, Ta CN. Evaluation and management of herpes zoster ophthalmicus. Am Fam Physician. 2002;66:1723–30.
22. Hunder GG, Bloch DA, Michel BA, Stevens MB, Arend WP, Calabrese LH, et al. The American College of Rheumatology 1990 criteria for the classification of giant cell arteritis. Arthritis Rheum. 1990;33:1122–8. https://doi.org/10.1002/art.1780330810.
23. Hayreh SS, Zimmerman MB, Kimura A, Sanon A. Central retinal artery occlusion. Retinal survival time. Exp Eye Res. 2004;78:723–36. https://doi.org/10.1016/S0014-4835(03)00214-8.
24. Nielsen NV. Treatment of acute occlusion of the retinal arteries. Acta Ophthalmol. 2009;57:1078–83. https://doi.org/10.1111/j.1755-3768.1979.tb00540.x.

Ear Pain + Cerumen Impaction

3

Emily Weeks

3.1 Introduction

Ear-related complaints are common presentations in both the primary care setting and in the emergency department. Ear pain, or otalgia, can be divided into primary otalgia, pain originating from the ear itself, and secondary otalgia, pain referred to the ear from another anatomic origin. The causes of otalgia can be further divided by age group, with infectious etiology being the most common overall, comprising the majority of diagnoses in the pediatric population and an increasing prevalence of secondary causes seen in the adult population [1]. The auricular and periauricular tissues receive sensory innervation from cranial nerves V, VII, IX, and X, as well as innervation from cervical roots C2 and C3, necessitating a broad differential in the approach to otalgia, including, but not limited to, those listed below [1].

3.2 Differential Diagnosis

Primary Otalgia

- Auricle
  - Auricular hematoma
  - Infectious—cellulitis, chondritis, and perichondritis
  - Herpes zoster oticus (Ramsay Hunt syndrome)
- External ear canal
  - Infectious—otitis externa, malignant otitis externa, and bullous myringitis
  - Cerumen impaction
  - Keratosis obturans
  - Foreign body

E. Weeks (✉)
University of Central Florida, Orlando, FL, USA

B. K. Desai et al. (eds.), *Primary Care for Emergency Physicians*,
https://doi.org/10.1007/978-3-031-64676-8_3

  - Neoplastic—tumor
- Middle and inner ear
  - Cholesteatoma
  - Eustachian tube dysfunction
  - Infectious—acute otitis media (AOM), otitis media with effusion (OME), labyrinthitis, and mastoiditis
  - Traumatic—tympanic membrane (TM) rupture, barotrauma, penetrating, and blunt

Secondary Otalgia

- Angina
- Bruxism
- Cervical spine arthritis
- Cricoarytenoid arthritis
- Lymphadenopathy/lymphadenitis (regional)
- Malignancy—oropharyngeal, laryngeal, esophageal, intracranial, and cervical spine
- Neuralgia—Bell's palsy and trigeminal neuralgia
- Oropharyngeal infections—dental caries, dental abscess, pharyngitis, tonsillitis, peritonsillar abscess, and retropharyngeal abscess
- Parotitis
- Sinusitis
- Temporomandibular joint (TMJ) syndrome
- Temporal (giant cell) arteritis
- Thyroiditis
- Vascular—carotid artery dissection and thoracic aortic aneurysm/dissection

3.3 History

As with any patient, a standard history of present illness should be elicited, including the context, duration, quality, severity, and progression of symptoms. Localization of pain (ask patient to point with one finger), radiation of pain, aggravating factors (positional symptoms, chewing), and patient demographics (age, smoking status) are key historical components. A thorough review of systems will help identify pertinent positives and negatives in working toward a differential diagnosis. History may be inherently limited in the large proportion of pediatric patients presenting with otalgia. Circumstances surrounding symptom onset can be important clues; for example, the history of a child playing with Legos preceding onset may raise concern for foreign body.

Symptoms that favor a primary cause of otalgia include otorrhea, tinnitus, hearing loss, and vertigo [1, 2]. With regard to secondary causes, inquire about associated rash, dental pain, and sore throat. Finally, in adults, risk factors for malignancy including smoking or chewing tobacco use and heavy alcohol consumption should be assessed. Timing of onset can vary between more acute causes of otalgia (otitis media, otitis externa, bullous myringitis, perichondritis) versus more insidious onset (neoplasm, tumor, cholesteatoma, and some secondary causes of otalgia). Severity of pain is not always indicative of severity of cause [1]. Dental abscess may present with severe pain, whereas malignancy may present with mild, dull pain.

Any history of traumatic injury, including penetrating trauma, acoustic trauma, or barotrauma (scuba diving, airplane flight, fireworks, or other blast injury), should raise concern for tympanic membrane rupture. Minor trauma, including blunt, burn, or even ear piercing, can be associated with cellulitis, chondritis, or perichondritis [2].

Infectious etiologies are much more likely to cause acute, continuous, gradually worsening pain and are often associated with a history of fever [2]. A history of brief, intermittent, sharp pain may suggest trigeminal neuralgia [1]. Association with chewing may suggest temporomandibular joint disorder, dental abscess, or dental caries [2]. In older patients, a history of pain worsened with range of motion of the neck could indicate cervical spine arthritis [2].

3.4 Physical Examination

A thorough physical examination should consist of otoscopic examination and evaluation of the auricle and postauricular region and should include examination of the head, oropharynx, nose, and neck. First, inspect the auricle for erythema, tenderness, or edema. Increased pain with traction on the pinna or pressure on the tragus suggests otitis externa or other pathology involving the external auditory canal [3].

Otoscopic evaluation, including of the external canal and tympanic membrane, may require cerumen removal, in the designated section below. Assess for pain, discharge, and narrowing of the external auditory canal associated with otitis externa and malignant otitis externa [3]. Inspect for masses consistent with malignancy, or "pearly mass" consistent with cholesteatoma [2]. A normal tympanic membrane should be mobile, intact, and translucent. The presence of a middle ear effusion with tympanic membrane bulging and erythema, with or without reduced mobility with insufflation, indicates likely acute otitis media [2]. Be sure to fully visualize the entire tympanic membrane to exclude perforation. Note that a previously normal tympanic membrane may take on an erythematous appearance immediately after any attempt at cerumen removal.

Next, evaluate for edema, warmth, and erythema over the mastoid process, effacement of the postauricular fold, and displacement of the pinna anteriorly and inferiorly, as these findings are indicative of mastoiditis [3]. Palpation of the temporomandibular joint (TMJ) on opening and closing of the mouth may reveal tenderness and crepitus, consistent with TMJ syndrome [3]. Particularly in the setting of trauma, and with the presence of hemotympanum, examination for Battle's signs (swelling, ecchymosis, and tenderness over the mastoid) should be undertaken, and consideration of further imaging for underlying basilar skull fracture given [2].

If the examination of the auricle and periauricular area is normal, careful evaluation for secondary causes of otalgia should be undertaken. Examination of the oropharynx should include visualization and palpation of dentition, especially molars, to evaluate for dental caries, infection, abscess, or impaction [3]. Pharyngitis, viral or bacterial, and tonsillitis are common causes of referred ear pain. Inspect and palpate the neck for masses, especially in patients with risk factors for malignancy, or tenderness consistent with lymphadenopathy/lymphadenitis. Anterior neck tenderness is suggestive of thyroiditis [2]. Range of motion assessment and palpation of the cervical spine can elicit findings suggesting arthritis or radiculopathy [2]. Tenderness in the temporal region suggesting giant cell arteritis in older patients or parotid tenderness and swelling indicative of parotitis should also be assessed [2].

3.5 Important Primary Otalgia Etiologies and Treatment

3.5.1 Acute Otitis Media

Acute otitis media (AOM) accounts for a significant number of visits to primary care offices and emergency departments and is the most frequent indication for antibiotic prescriptions in children [4]. The peak incidence occurs between the ages of 6 and 18 months [4]. Daycare attendance, family history of AOM, air pollution (including exposure to tobacco smoke), and lack of breastfeeding are factors associated with increased risk [4].

Acute otitis media is most commonly preceded by a viral upper respiratory illness. Inflammation and increased respiratory secretions result in obstruction of the Eustachian tube(s), leading to pooling of secretions in the middle ear, and bacterial and/or viral growth. *Streptococcus pneumoniae* (~45% of bacterial isolates), non-typeable *Haemophilus influenzae* (~45%), and *Moraxella catarrhalis* (~10%) are most common bacterial pathogens [4]. *S. pneumoniae* once accounted for a much larger proportion of infections, but the use of polyvalent pneumococcal conjugate vaccine has resulted in a marked decline in its prevalence in middle ear isolates [4]. Respiratory syncytial virus, influenza, and adenoviruses are also associated with the diagnosis.

Diagnosis of AOM requires both evidence of middle ear inflammation and presence of tympanic membrane bulging or otorrhea (not due to otitis externa) [5]. Inflammation is commonly manifested as erythema of the tympanic membrane, otalgia, or fever [5]. A bulging, cloudy, or erythematous tympanic membrane, with lack of tympanic membrane mobility on pneumatic otoscopy, is very strongly suggestive of the diagnosis [6].

Treatment of AOM includes analgesia and consideration of antibiotic therapy. While immediate initiation of antibiotic therapy was once routine, recent guidelines have advocated for consideration of a 24–48-h watchful waiting period prior to antibiotic initiation in lower-risk patients and immediate antibiotic initiation in higher-risk patients. In children 6 months and older, antibiotic therapy should be initiated immediately in AOM with otorrhea, severe symptoms (toxic-appearing child, otalgia >48 h, fever 39 °C (102.2 °F) or higher), bilateral AOM, and patients without reliable follow-up [7]. Deferred treatment, or watchful waiting, may be considered in unilateral AOM without otorrhea or bilateral AOM in those over 2 years old with onset of symptoms <48 h prior, absence of severe symptoms, and guaranteed follow-up within 48–72 h [7].

First-line treatment of AOM is amoxicillin 80–90 mg/kg/day in two divided doses [5]. Amoxicillin/clavulanate (Augmentin) should be the initial antibiotic for children who have taken amoxicillin for AOM within 30 days or for those with purulent conjunctivitis [5]. In patients with non-anaphylactic penicillin hypersensitivity, cefdinir is the first-line treatment of AOM. Azithromycin may be used if cephalosporins are not tolerated or in anaphylactic penicillin hypersensitivity [5].

Treatment failure is defined as severe AOM symptoms not resolving within 48–72 h of treatment initiation, or recurrent AOM within 30 days, and most commonly results from beta-lactamase-producing *H. influenzae* or *M. catarrhalis* [5]. Duration of treatment is based on age and symptom severity. A 10-day treatment course is recommended for children less than 2 years old, patients with severe symptoms, and patients with prior treatment failure. A 7-day treatment course is recommended in non-severe cases in children over the age of 2 [5].

Referral to otolaryngology is warranted in persistent treatment failure, three or more episodes of AOM within 6 months, or four episodes within 1 year (at least one in the preceding 6 months) [5].

Recognized sequelae of AOM include conductive hearing loss, balance difficulties, tympanic membrane perforation, cholesteatoma formation, and progressive extension of infection to contiguous structures (potentially resulting in mastoiditis, meningitis/intracerebral abscess, and septic lateral or cavernous sinus thrombosis) [6].

3.5.2 Otitis Media with Effusion

Middle ear effusion is a persistent finding in many patients with a recent diagnosis of AOM, regardless of whether antibiotics were initially prescribed, with a prevalence of 70% at 2 weeks and 10% at 3 months [8]. Eustachian tube dysfunction, tobacco exposure/abuse, and chronic sinus disease can also lead to chronic effusion [8]. Symptoms can include diminished hearing and a sense of aural fullness. Nonurgent ENT referral is indicated if an effusion has been present for >3 months, as there is concern for development of permanent hearing impairment in children. Antibiotics, antihistamines, and decongestants are *not* indicated [6].

3.5.3 Acute Otitis Externa

Acute otitis externa (AOE), also known as swimmer's ear, refers to inflammation and infection of the external ear canal. Causes of AOE can include allergic and dermatologic, but infectious (bacterial infection) is the most common cause. It can occur in all age groups but is more common in children and young adults [9]. It can occur year-round but is more common in the summer, due to increased heat and humidity, as well as increased water-related activities [10]. Swimming is the most common risk factor, with others including anatomic abnormalities, canal obstruction, compromised epithelial integrity (earplug use, hearing aid use), and certain dermatologic conditions (eczema, psoriasis, seborrhea) [9]. Classic presentation of AOE is rapid onset of otalgia within 48 h, with symptoms of ear canal inflammation (ear pain, itching, sense of fullness), and signs of canal inflammation (pinna or tragus tenderness or diffuse canal edema or redness) [11]. Other associated symptoms may include otorrhea, concurrent otitis media, tympanic membrane rupture, and local lymphadenitis [11].

The most common bacterial pathogens identified in AOE are *Pseudomonas aeruginosa* (20–60%) and *Staphylococcus aureus* (10–70%), most often occurring as a polymicrobial infection [11]. Fungal involvement is less common in primary AOE but should be considered in chronic otitis externa, or treatment failure.

Treatment of AOE includes gentle cleaning of debris, analgesia, and topical therapy. A variety of topical treatment options exist. Steroids have been shown effective in reducing pain and inflammation, and several antibiotic/glucocorticoid preparations are commercially available [6]. In patients with a severely occluded ear canal, an ear wick moistened with antibiotic drops may be placed in order to facilitate medication delivery. Patients using ear wicks or with severe inflammation and high-risk groups for development of malignant otitis externa should also have close otolaryngology follow-up [1].

In treatment consideration, isolated AOE should be distinguished from AOE with concomitant acute otitis media (AOM). In uncomplicated, isolated AOE, topical treatment should be the initial therapy unless there is associated AOM, extension of cellulitis to the outer ear canal, or an immunocompromised host, all of which warrant systemic/oral antibiotic therapy [11]. When the patient has a known or suspected tympanic membrane perforation, or presence of tympanostomy tube(s), non-ototoxic topical preparations should be used. Topical preparations include antibiotic (polymyxin B, quinolones, aminoglycosides (ototoxic)), steroid (hydrocortisone or dexamethasone), or low-pH antiseptic (replication of *P. aeruginosa* and *S. aureus* is inhibited at pH <6) [11]. Neomycin is an aminoglycoside often prescribed in conjunction with a steroid as first-line therapy for acute otitis externa. Advantages include low cost and efficacy compared to other antibiotic/steroid combinations [11]. Due to concern for aminoglycoside ototoxicity if introduced to the middle ear, preparations containing this agent should be avoided if tympanic membrane rupture may be present or in the presence of tympanostomy tubes. Neomycin can also directly cause skin irritation, complicating recovery for affected patients. Fluoroquinolone drops (ofloxacin or ciprofloxacin) are generally preferred due to lower concern for ototoxicity and inflammation [6].

Common topical preparations include acetic acid 2.0% solution (with or without hydrocortisone 1.0%), ciprofloxacin 0.2% with hydrocortisone 1.0%, and ciprofloxacin 0.3% with dexamethasone 0.1%, which do not have generic alternatives and therefore can be cost prohibitive, neomycin/polymyxin B/hydrocortisone, and ofloxacin 0.3% [11]. There was no significant difference in clinical outcomes between antiseptic and antimicrobial preparations, quinolone and non-quinolone antibiotic, or antimicrobial alone and antimicrobial with steroid combination [11].

Pitfall: Failure of acute otitis externa to resolve within 2–3 weeks despite adherence to appropriate treatment strongly suggests the diagnosis of necrotizing otitis externa [12].

3.5.4 Necrotizing (Malignant) Otitis Externa

Extension of otitis externa infection to structures beyond the soft tissues of the external ear canal is termed necrotizing (malignant) otitis externa. Risk factors include diabetes mellitus, immunocompromised state, and elderly age [12]. Pseudomonas is the most frequently associated pathogen, although recently MRSA has been increasingly associated with the condition [13]. Fungal etiologies are rare but should be considered in severely immunocompromised patients, especially patients with poorly controlled diabetes and HIV/AIDS (especially CD4 counts <50/mm^3) and those undergoing chemotherapy/radiation [12, 13]. Decreased vascular supply from microvascular disease (diabetes mellitus) and decreased immune response/polymorphonuclear cell function (immunosuppressed state) can lead to extension of infection to cartilaginous skeleton of ear and eventually to the temporal bone via Santorini's fissures, causing osteitis of the base of the skull [12]. Hallmarks of extension of infection include granulation tissue in the bone-cartilage junction of the external auditory canal (pathognomonic), pain out of proportion, cervical lymphadenopathy, trismus (in temporomandibular joint involvement), masseter muscle irritation, and eventually cranial nerve palsies [12]. The tympanic membrane, when visualized, often appears normal.

Cranial nerve involvement, most commonly CN VII (facial nerve) within the temporal bone, results from compression and bony destruction as infection extends through the foramina and local secretion of neurotoxins. Cranial nerve involvement is associated with a poor prognosis, as it indicates intracranial extension of infection, and death most commonly results from intracranial complications (dural sinus thrombosis, meningitis, intracranial abscess, internal carotid artery pseudoaneurysm) [12, 14].

Diagnosis of necrotizing otitis externa begins with a high clinical suspicion in patients with otitis externa and significant risk factors for extension of infection, otitis externa refractory to treatment, and severe otalgia out of proportion to physical exam, especially at night [12]. Laboratory testing commonly reveals an elevation in erythrocyte sedimentation rate (ESR), and white blood cell count, and should include glucose, creatinine levels, and canal secretion cultures, if possible, prior to antibiotic initiation. Imaging modalities, such as computed tomographic (CT) scan, technetium Tc99m bone scanning, and gallium citrate ^{67}Ga scintigraphy, may be used to confirm extension to bony structures [12]. One third of bone mineralization must be lost before radiologic changes become evident on CT; therefore, pathology may be late to appear on imaging [12]. Macrophages and reticuloendothelial system cells absorb ^{67}Ga, making this more sensitive for ongoing infection and useful for early initial diagnosis, when available [12].

Treatment of malignant otitis externa is multifaceted and includes aggressive management of underlying immunosuppression when present, strict glucose control in diabetes mellitus, long-term systemic antibiotic therapy, and sometimes surgical intervention. Antibiotic therapy with antipseudomonal activity (aminoglycosides, piperacillin-tazobactam, ceftazidime, cefepime, and sometimes imipenem) should be continued for at least 4 weeks, and oral antibiotic options are limited secondary to resistance, especially in fluoroquinolones [12]. Otolaryngology should be involved early, for consideration of debridement, and abscess drainage, and to ensure adequate follow-up [12].

3.5.5 Acute Mastoiditis

Mastoiditis is a suppurative infection of the air cells of the mastoid process. Historically the most common complication of acute otitis media (AOM), incidence of acute mastoiditis has decreased with increased early AOM recognition and antibiotic treatment, although acute mastoiditis may still be the first presentation of AOM [15]. Children, especially those under 2 years of age, are at increased risk, due to increased prevalence of middle ear infections compared to adults. Recurrent AOM and delayed antibiotic treatment are also associated with higher risk. Acute mastoiditis may be further divided, according to stage, into acute mastoiditis with periostitis (purulent material in the mastoid cavities without destruction of bony septa) and acute mastoid osteitis (destruction of the bony septa between air cells) [15].

The mastoid, a division of the temporal bone, begins as the antrum, connected to the middle ear by a narrow channel, and becomes pneumatized as a child grows [16]. In acute otitis media, the middle ear (connected to the mastoid air spaces) becomes inflamed, with associated fluid collection. Progression of inflammation along the respiratory epithelium lining the mastoid air cells, along with accumulation of purulent material in the mastoid cavities, can lead to increased mastoid pressure and destruction of bony septa (acute mastoiditis) [16]. If not treated, abscess formation may occur, with extension into adjacent structures.

Diagnosis of acute mastoiditis in children can be made clinically in the majority of cases, when characteristic findings of postauricular tenderness, erythema, swelling or mass, loss of postauricular crease and protrusion of the auricle/pinna, otalgia (may only present as irritability or ear tugging in young children/infants), and fever are present [17]. Other commonly associated symptoms include lethargy/malaise (96%), abnormal tympanic membrane (82%), and fever (76%) [17]. Tympanic membrane (TM) evaluation may reveal bulging, effusion, or perforation, but TM is often unable to be visualized secondary to external canal inflammation [17]. The absence of AOM diagnosis does not exclude acute mastoiditis.

Laboratory studies in acute mastoiditis may include normal/elevated white blood cell count and elevation of erythrocyte sedimentation rate or C-reactive protein, although these findings are nonspecific [18]. Imaging is not necessary for diagnosis, especially in children, but CT with contrast or MRI with gadolinium contrast may be utilized in the absence of characteristic findings and is especially helpful when intracranial complications are suspected. In children, the most common CT findings include mastoid opacification/clouding, which is also a common finding in AOM and in isolation is not diagnostic of acute mastoiditis [18]. Findings diagnostic of acute mastoiditis include loss of definition of bony septa, destruction or irregularity of mastoid cortex, and subperiosteal abscess [6, 18].

Pathogenesis of acute mastoiditis is similar to that of acute otitis media, with *S. pneumoniae, S. pyogenes*, and *H. influenzae* most commonly isolated and *S. aureus*, *F. necrophorum,* and *P. aeruginosa* also recognized as causative organisms [19, 20].

Treatment and management of acute mastoiditis involves systemic antibiotic therapy, early otolaryngology consultation, and possible neurosurgical consultation in cases of intracranial complications. Myringotomy (with or without tympanostomy tube placement for middle ear drainage) and fluid culture can help guide antibiotic selection. Empiric antibiotic therapy considerations include age, recent antibiotic use/treatment, and history of recurrent otitis media. With high incidence of *S. pneumoniae*, sensitivity to cephalosporins has been shown superior compared to penicillins [21]. Initially, broad-spectrum antibiotics with coverage for MRSA and pseudomonas should be initiated [18, 21, 22]. Although antibiotic therapy is highly variable, especially among children, most common regimens include a cephalosporin (ceftazidime or cefepime) or piperacillin-tazobactam and vancomycin [18, 22]. Systemic intravenous antibiotics should be continued for at least 7–10 days prior to transition to oral antibiotics, with at least 4 weeks of antibiotic treatment time [21]. Vancomycin should be included for all patients with possible MRSA or clinical signs of sepsis. Antipseudomonal coverage is especially important in patients with recent antibiotic use and/or recurrent AOM. Cephalosporins provide better central nervous system (CNS) penetration in patients with possible intracranial complications including meningitis [21–23]. Surgical debridement may be required in the absence of appropriate response to antibiotics [23].

Pitfall: If inadequately treated, mastoiditis can progress to osteomyelitis of the petrous bone (petrositis), resulting in sixth and seventh cranial nerve palsies, permanent hearing impairment, meningitis, intracranial abscess, and venous sinus thrombosis [17].

Pitfall: The possibility of masked (subacute) mastoiditis in patients with AOM unresponsive to antibiotics should be considered. In such patients, complications of mastoiditis such as those listed above may arise without classic signs and symptoms of mastoiditis [24].

3.5.6 Foreign Bodies

Aural foreign bodies can present with a variety of chief complaints in both the emergency department and primary care setting. Occasionally, a more immediate presentation occurs in the setting of known foreign body, but presentation and diagnosis are often delayed as most events are unobserved, symptoms are nonspecific, or patients may be asymptomatic [25]. Most patients with foreign bodies are children [25]. Foreign body shape, location, and material have important implications in successful removal. The most cited foreign bodies include beads, insects, pebbles, and beans [26]. Foreign bodies may become impacted at the bony cartilaginous junction, the narrowest portion of the external auditory canal [25]. Attempts at foreign body removal must be taken with caution and preparation, as foreign bodies may be pushed further into the canal, increasing risk of tympanic membrane damage. Optimal visualization, a cooperative patient, adequate preparation, and a graspable (soft and irregular, e.g., foam, rubber, paper, vegetable material) foreign body with appropriate tools yield the best chance of removal without subspecialist referral [25]. Indications for subspecialist removal include need for sedation, external canal or tympanic membrane trauma, ungraspable object (hard, spherical, e.g., beads/pebbles/popcorn kernels), sharp objects (e.g., glass), objects abutting TM, or multiple unsuccessful attempts at removal [25]. The highest success rates occur on first removal attempt and decrease markedly on subsequent attempts [26].

Techniques for foreign body removal include water irrigation, forceps removal (most commonly alligator forceps), cerumen loops, right-angle ball hooks, and suction catheters. In the case of live insects, when the TM is intact and not perforated, alcohol, 2% lidocaine, or mineral oil should be used in the canal prior to removal to ensure the insect is no longer moving [25]. Irrigation should be avoided in button batteries as contents can lead to liquefaction tissue necrosis [27].

3.5.7 Traumatic Tympanic Membrane Perforation

Traumatic perforation of the tympanic membrane may arise from blunt trauma (most common), barotrauma, blast injury, or penetrating trauma [28]. Patients are most commonly adults, with highest prevalence in young males, and presenting symptoms include fullness, tinnitus, and conductive hearing loss [28]. Although management has historically been controversial, water precautions alone and spontaneous healing have up to 95% success rates [28]. Myringoplasty may be indicated if spontaneous healing does not occur within 3–6 months, in the absence of secondary infection. Time to healing was related to size of perforation, with very large perforations (involving 80% or more of the area of the tympanic membrane) rarely healing spontaneously [28]. Appropriate supportive care results in improved healing compared with early surgical repair, and the majority of cases result in spontaneous healing without need for further surgical intervention [28].

Pitfall: Severe vertigo following a ruptured tympanic membrane suggests the presence of a perilymphatic fistula or rupture of the round window. In this scenario, urgent ENT consultation is necessary [29].

3.5.8 Cerumen Impaction

Cerumen (earwax) production is a normal, protective mechanism for the external ear canal. Occasionally, cerumen may become impacted or form an abnormal accumulation with or without complete obstruction, secondary to failure of normal clearance mechanisms or due to mechanical attempts at clearance. Cerumen impaction is a common issue, with a prevalence of approximately 10% in children (in which case limited evaluation of the tympanic membrane is possible) and much higher rates (up to >50%) noted in elderly and developmentally delayed patients [30, 31]. Cerumen removal should be considered when canal impaction becomes symptomatic (hearing loss, pain, irritation, tinnitus), when accumulation does not allow for assessment of the external canal or tympanic membrane, and in patients who may be unable to fully communicate their symptoms (elderly, nonverbal, young children) [31].

Patient-specific modifying factors including age, medical history, medications, surgical history, and ability to cooperate with procedure are important factors for consideration prior to removal. History of hepatic failure or cirrhosis, coagulopathy (hemophilia, von Willebrand's disease, thrombocytopenia), and antiplatelet/anticoagulant use have an increased risk of bleeding associated with cerumen removal, and attempts at mechanical removal should be taken gently, or patients referred to subspecialists [31]. Patients with immunosuppression (malignancy, chemotherapy, uncontrolled diabetes) carry a higher risk of otitis externa post-procedure, which may progress rapidly to malignant otitis externa, making them higher risk for complications [31]. Patients with history of head/neck radiation may require additional care in debridement as increased risk of osteoradionecrosis is associated with external canal injury [31].

Various methods for cerumen impaction removal may be used, and most can be easily performed in the outpatient clinic setting. The three most widely utilized methods include cerumenolytic agents, irrigation, and manual removal via instrumentation; methods may be used alone or in conjunction with one another [32].

Cerumenolytic or softening agents include topical preparations which may be oil-based (e.g., almond oil, mineral oil), water-based (e.g., acetic acid, hydrogen peroxide, sodium bicarbonate, water, or saline), or non-water/oil-based (e.g., carbamide peroxide, propylene glycol) [33]. Topical preparations should not be used if tympanostomy tubes are present or in cases where tympanic membrane may not be intact. A 2010 systematic review of 26 clinical trials concluded that the use of softeners overall led to increased clearance compared to methods without softener use, but no single softener consistently outperformed others [33]. Most preparations are applied for a period of 15–30 min, after which attempts at removal may be made [34]. Effectiveness of irrigation and mechanical removal was equivocal [33].

Irrigation may be used alone or after cerumenolytic treatment. Methods for irrigation include manual irrigation with a syringe (most common), jet irrigators, or several electronic irrigators marketed for this use. Irrigation fluid (water or normal saline) should be close to body temperature to prevent caloric stimulation and vertigo, and irrigation should be directed toward the superior aspect of the canal to minimize direct pressure on the tympanic membrane [35]. Frequent reassessment of the external canal and tympanic membrane for clearance and possible complications should occur. Although rare (1/1000 attempts), tympanic membrane perforation is considered a major complication [33]. Irrigation should not be performed if tympanostomy tubes are present or in cases where tympanic membrane may not be intact.

Mechanical removal may be faster and sometimes more safe, especially with nonintact tympanic membrane, systemic illness, and abnormal ear canal anatomy. It requires a more cooperative patient and additional clinical skill compared to other methods [33]. Mechanical removal can be achieved with a variety of instruments including curettes, loops, spoons, alligator forceps, and suction tips. Adequate visualization is of the utmost importance to minimize complications and may be obtained using an otoscope with speculum, headlight, or binocular microscope [33].

Pitfall: Tap water canal irrigation of diabetics and the immunocompromised, particularly if an abrasion is present, may result in malignant otitis externa. Consider the use of acidifying ear drops post-procedure if this method is utilized, and provide explicit return precautions for the development of symptoms of otitis externa [33].

Pitfall: The use of cotton-tipped applicators to attempt removal of cerumen often leads to worsened impaction and can result in infection and rupture of the tympanic membrane. Patients should be counseled to avoid this technique.

References

1. Neilan RE, Roland PS. Otalgia. Med Clin N Am. 2010;94(5):961–71. https://doi.org/10.1016/j.mcna.2010.05.004.
2. Earwood JS, Rogers TS, Rathjen NA. Ear pain: diagnosing common and uncommon causes. Am Fam Physician. 2018;97(1):20–7.
3. Ely JW, Hansen MR, Clark EC. Diagnosis of ear pain. Am Fam Physician. 2008;77(5):621–8.
4. Coker TR, Chan LS, Newberry SJ, et al. Diagnosis, microbial epidemiology, and antibiotic treatment of acute otitis media in children: a systematic review. JAMA. 2010;304(19):2161–9. https://doi.org/10.1001/jama.2010.1651.
5. Lieberthal AS, Carroll AE, Chonmaitree T, et al. The diagnosis and management of acute otitis media [published correction appears in pediatrics. 2014 Feb;133(2):346. Dosage error in article text]. Pediatrics. 2013;131(3):e964–99. https://doi.org/10.1542/peds.2012-3488.
6. Conover K. Earache. Emerg Med Clin N Am. 2013;31(2):413–42. https://doi.org/10.1016/j.emc.2013.02.001.
7. Gaddey HL, Wright MT, Nelson TN. Otitis media: rapid evidence review. Am Fam Physician. 2019;100(6):350–6.
8. Teele DW, Klein JO, Rosner BA. Epidemiology of otitis media in children. Ann Otol Rhinol Laryngol Suppl. 1980;89(3 Pt 2):5–6. https://doi.org/10.1177/00034894800890s304.
9. Jackson EA, Geer K. Acute otitis externa: rapid evidence review. Am Fam Physician. 2023;107(2):145–51.
10. Beers SL, Abramo TJ. Otitis externa review. Pediatr Emerg Care. 2004;20(4):250–6. https://doi.org/10.1097/01.pec.0000121246.99242.f5.
11. Rosenfeld RM, Schwartz SR, Cannon CR, et al. Clinical practice guideline: acute otitis externa [published correction appears in Otolaryngol Head Neck Surg. 2014 Mar;150(3):504] [published correction appears in Otolaryngol Head Neck Surg. 2014 Mar;150(3):504]. Otolaryngol Head Neck Surg. 2014;150(1 Suppl):S1–S24. https://doi.org/10.1177/0194599813517083.

12. Handzel O, Halperin D. Necrotizing (malignant) external otitis. Am Fam Physician. 2003;68(2):309–12.
13. Hobson CE, Moy JD, Byers KE, Raz Y, Hirsch BE, McCall AA. Malignant otitis externa: evolving pathogens and implications for diagnosis and treatment. Otolaryngol Head Neck Surg. 2014;151(1):112–6. https://doi.org/10.1177/0194599814528301.
14. Schwarz GA, Blumenkrantz MJ, Sundmäker WL. Neurologic complications of malignant external otitis. Neurology. 1971;21(11):1077–84. https://doi.org/10.1212/wnl.21.11.1077.
15. Maranhão A, Andrade J, Godofredo V, Matos R, Penido N. Epidemiology of intratemporal complications of otitis media. Int Arch Otorhinolaryngol. 2014;18(2):178–83. https://doi.org/10.1055/s-0033-1364172.
16. Lin HW, Shargorodsky J, Gopen Q. Clinical strategies for the management of acute mastoiditis in the pediatric population. Clin Pediatr (Phila). 2010;49(2):110–5. https://doi.org/10.1177/0009922809344349.
17. van den Aardweg MT, Rovers MM, de Ru JA, Albers FW, Schilder AG. A systematic review of diagnostic criteria for acute mastoiditis in children. Otol Neurotol. 2008;29(6):751–7. https://doi.org/10.1097/MAO.0b013e31817f736b.
18. Stähelin-Massik J, Podvinec M, Jakscha J, et al. Mastoiditis in children: a prospective, observational study comparing clinical presentation, microbiology, computed tomography, surgical findings and histology. Eur J Pediatr. 2008;167(5):541–8. https://doi.org/10.1007/s00431-007-0549-1.
19. Mansour T, Yehudai N, Tobia A, et al. Acute mastoiditis: 20 years of experience with a uniform management protocol. Int J Pediatr Otorhinolaryngol. 2019;125:187–91. https://doi.org/10.1016/j.ijporl.2019.07.014.
20. Luntz M, Brodsky A, Nusem S, et al. Acute mastoiditis—the antibiotic era: a multicenter study. Int J Pediatr Otorhinolaryngol. 2001;57(1):1–9. https://doi.org/10.1016/s0165-5876(00)00425-0.
21. Cassano P, Ciprandi G, Passali D. Acute mastoiditis in children. Acta Biomed. 2020;91(1-S):54–9. Published 2020 Feb 17. https://doi.org/10.23750/abm.v91i1-S.9259.
22. Edwards S, Kumar S, Lee S, Pali BL, Marek RL, Dutta A. Epidemiology and variability in management of acute mastoiditis in children. Am J Otolaryngol. 2022;43(5):103520. https://doi.org/10.1016/j.amjoto.2022.103520.
23. Geva A, Oestreicher-Kedem Y, Fishman G, Landsberg R, DeRowe A. Conservative management of acute mastoiditis in children. Int J Pediatr Otorhinolaryngol. 2008;72(5):629–34. https://doi.org/10.1016/j.ijporl.2008.01.013.
24. Holt GR, Gates GA. Masked mastoiditis. Laryngoscope. 1983;93(8):1034–7. https://doi.org/10.1288/00005537-198308000-00011.
25. Heim SW, Maughan KL. Foreign bodies in the ear, nose, and throat. Am Fam Physician. 2007;76(8):1185–9.
26. Schulze SL, Kerschner J, Beste D. Pediatric external auditory canal foreign bodies: a review of 698 cases. Otolaryngol Head Neck Surg. 2002;127(1):73–8. https://doi.org/10.1067/mhn.2002.126724.
27. Balbani AP, Sanchez TG, Butugan O, et al. Ear and nose foreign body removal in children. Int J Pediatr Otorhinolaryngol. 1998;46(1–2):37–42. https://doi.org/10.1016/s0165-5876(98)00118-9.
28. Sagiv D, Migirov L, Glikson E, et al. Traumatic perforation of the tympanic membrane: a review of 80 cases. J Emerg Med. 2018;54(2):186–90. https://doi.org/10.1016/j.jemermed.2017.09.018.
29. Maitland CG. Perilymphatic fistula. Curr Neurol Neurosci Rep. 2001;1(5):486–91. https://doi.org/10.1007/s11910-001-0111-x.
30. Roeser RJ, Ballachanda BB. Physiology, pathophysiology, and anthropology/epidemiology of human earcanal secretions. J Am Acad Audiol. 1997;8(6):391–400.
31. Michaudet C, Malaty J. Cerumen impaction: diagnosis and management. Am Fam Physician. 2018;98(8):525–9.

32. Schwartz SR, Magit AE, Rosenfeld RM, et al. Clinical practice guideline (update): Earwax (Cerumen Impaction) [published correction appears in Otolaryngol Head Neck Surg. 2017 Sep;157(3):539]. Otolaryngol Head Neck Surg. 2017;156(1_suppl):S1–S29. https://doi.org/10.1177/0194599816671491.
33. Clegg AJ, Loveman E, Gospodarevskaya E, et al. The safety and effectiveness of different methods of earwax removal: a systematic review and economic evaluation. Health Technol Assess. 2010;14(28):1–192. https://doi.org/10.3310/hta14280.
34. Burton MJ, Dorée CJ. Ear drops for the removal of ear wax. Cochrane Database Syst Rev. 2003;3:CD004400. https://doi.org/10.1002/14651858.CD004400.
35. Roland PS, Smith TL, Schwartz SR, et al. Clinical practice guideline: cerumen impaction. Otolaryngol Head Neck Surg. 2008;139(3 Suppl 2):S1–S21. https://doi.org/10.1016/j.otohns.2008.06.026.

Sore Throat, Dental Pain, and Other Oral Issues

4

Alpa Desai

4.1 Introduction

Chief complaints such as "sore throat" and "dental pain" are some of the most common encountered by primary care and emergency physicians. In the vast majority of cases, the diagnosis is quite benign, which can lull the clinician into a false sense of security when evaluating patients with these complaints. However, the differential ranges from routine self-limited etiologies to immediately life-threatening conditions. Furthermore, the availability of emergent dental consultation is often quite limited during much of the week, while dental emergencies occur continuously. Therefore, the clinician must possess a solid knowledge base with respect to the evaluation and management of these conditions.

4.2 History

The history obtained in patients presenting with oropharyngeal complaints should rapidly assess for any red flags for impending respiratory failure. A change in voice (particularly a "hot potato" voice), dyspnea, submandibular swelling, and rapidly worsening symptoms are red flags for a potential obstructive process such as a deep space infection that may mandate immediate intervention.

Once immediate evidence of an obstructive process has been excluded, further historical detail can be obtained to narrow the differential. In addition to the standard elements of the patient history that should be elicited for a complaint of pain in any region of the body, assess for associated symptoms including fever, malaise, congestion, rhinorrhea, and cough. The presence of any urogenital symptoms is

A. Desai (✉)
Department of Community Health and Family Medicine, University of Florida College of Medicine, Gainesville, FL, USA

B. K. Desai et al. (eds.), *Primary Care for Emergency Physicians*,
https://doi.org/10.1007/978-3-031-64676-8_4

relevant if there exists concern for gonorrheal pharyngitis or oral herpes simplex infection.

Past medical history should focus on immunocompromising conditions (including splenectomy), which may predispose to rapid propagation of infection to a potentially life-threatening process. If oral abscess drainage is being considered, ask about any history of cardiac conditions such as a valve replacement or congenital defect that requires endocarditis prophylaxis. Immunization history is of importance when epiglottitis or diphtheria is in the differential. Finally, assess for risk factors for development of oropharyngeal cancer, including past or present use of chewing tobacco and/or smoking, alcohol abuse, family history of malignancies, and occupational exposures.

4.3 Physical

The initial step in the physical examination of any patient with symptoms affecting the oropharynx should be evaluation for any evidence of respiratory distress (tripod posture, cyanosis, inability to handle secretions), which will require immediate securing of the airway and ventilator support due to the potential for a progressive obstructive process. Following this, a systematic approach to the physical exam should be employed.

- External exam
  - "Hot potato" voice (*red flag): deep space infections
  - Submandibular swelling (*red flag): Ludwig's angina
  - Trismus (*red flag): deep space infections
  - Cervical lymphadenopathy: numerous infectious/inflammatory processes, malignancy
  - Facial asymmetry: odontogenic infection/abscess, sialoadenitis
  - Lip swelling: if atraumatic (*red flag), angioedema; traumatic, hematoma
- Internal exam
  - Posterior oropharynx
    - Tonsillar asymmetry (*red flag): peritonsillar abscess
    - Uvular edema (*red flag): uvulitis
    - Pseudomembrane (*red flag): diphtheria
    - Erythema
    - Exudates
  - Tongue
    - Protrusion/displacement (*red flag): Ludwig's angina, angioedema
    - Swelling (*red flag): angioedema
    - Discoloration
  - Teeth/gums
    - Caries
    - Dental fractures
    - Tenderness: tenderness of teeth to percussion suggests pulpitis/abscess

    - Tenderness of gums
    - Fluctuance
  - Masses (*red flag): malignancy
- Ear exam
  - Evaluate for acute otitis media, otitis externa, and other potential sources of referred pain

4.4 Specific Etiologies

4.4.1 Sore Throat

4.4.1.1 Viral Pharyngitis

- Viral pharyngitis is the most common cause of sore throat.
- Symptoms are typically associated with a progression of other upper respiratory infection symptoms including congestion, rhinorrhea, and cough.
- Physical exam findings are of limited utility in distinguishing viral pharyngitis from a bacterial etiology.
- A variety of viral pathogens have been implicated, including influenza, Epstein-Barr (see below), cytomegalovirus, rhinovirus, and adenoviruses. In the vast majority of cases, identification of a specific etiologic indicated is unnecessary, as there is no specific treatment and the illness is self-limited.
- If influenza is suspected and the patient has been symptomatic for less than 48 h, consider treatment with oseltamivir.
- Testing may also be considered for mononucleosis if suspected clinically (see below).
- In patients at high risk for human immunodeficiency virus infection, consider the possibility of the acute retroviral syndrome.
- Otherwise, in the vast majority of patients, treatment is purely supportive.
- Nonsteroidal anti-inflammatory drugs and acetaminophen are mainstays of therapy.
- Adult patients can alternatively use aspirin-containing products.
- Formal studies regarding the efficacy of topical treatments are lacking.
- Numerous over-the-counter preparations are available, including lozenges containing benzocaine or menthol and sprays containing phenol.
- Patients should be counseled to avoid grossly excessive use of products containing benzocaine due to the theoretical possibility of inducing methemoglobinemia.
- All patients should be encouraged to maintain adequate hydration [1].

4.4.1.2 Streptococcal Pharyngitis

- Streptococcal pharyngitis is a common, easily treatable etiology of sore throat.
- The incidence is highest in children aged 5–15, although adults are also commonly infected.

- In addition to sore throat and dysphagia, patients with strep pharyngitis also commonly complain of fever, headache, and abdominal pain.
- The presence of cough, rhinorrhea, congestion, and conjunctivitis argues against the diagnosis.
- On exam, palatal petechiae, pharyngeal erythema, tonsillar exudates, tender anterior cervical lymphadenopathy, and scarlet fever (an erythematous, finely papular rash which spares the face) may be noted [2].

4.4.1.3 Centor Criteria

- The Centor criteria are a widely used scoring system to estimate the probability of a diagnosis of streptococcal pharyngitis.
- One point is assigned for the presence of each of the following factors:
  - Fever >38 °C.
  - Tender anterior cervical lymph nodes.
  - Presence of tonsillar exudates.
  - Absence of cough.
- A score of 0 is associated with a likelihood of streptococcal pharyngitis of approximately 2.5%, while a score of 4 has been associated with a >50% probability of infection.
- Guidelines issued by several professional societies concur that in a patient with a Centor score of 0, no further testing or treatment is necessary.
- Many authorities agree that in those with a score of 1 or 2, a rapid strep test with subsequent culture if negative is reasonable, while the use of additional testing in those with scores of 3–4 is controversial [1].
  - The sensitivity of rapid streptococcal testing is quoted between 70 and 90%, with excellent specificity [2].
  - Patients with negative rapid strep testing should have a throat culture obtained.
- Without treatment, streptococcal pharyngitis is self-limiting, with improvement in symptoms expected within 1 week.
- However, as streptococcal pharyngitis can result in rheumatic fever and post-streptococcal glomerulonephritis, all US guidelines call for treatment in patients with a positive rapid strep test or culture.
  - Acceptable treatment regimens include either oral penicillin VK for 10 days or one-time IM benzathine penicillin G.
  - Cephalosporins, azithromycin, erythromycin, and clindamycin are acceptable alternatives in penicillin-allergic patients, depending on the severity of the reaction.
- Supportive care for sore throat, as detailed above for viral pharyngitis, is also appropriate.

4.4.1.4 Mononucleosis

- Infectious mononucleosis is caused by the Epstein-Barr virus, which is transmitted though oral secretions.
- Children as well as adults can be affected, with younger patients typically having a less severe course [3].

- The condition typically presents with flu-like symptoms, including prominent sore throat, fatigue, headache, and fever.
- A prolonged duration of symptoms is a particular clue to the diagnosis, which can be difficult to differentiate from other causes of sore throat.
- Physical exam findings include marked anterior and posterior cervical lymphadenopathy, hepatomegaly, and splenomegaly.
- A maculopapular rash is sometimes observed, typically following the use of an antibiotic due to presumed earlier diagnosis of bacterial pharyngitis.
- The monospot test is commonly used to confirm the diagnosis.
- However, as this test relies on the presence of antibodies to Epstein-Barr virus, false-negative testing can be observed early in the disease course.
- Treatment is supportive, with the use of NSAIDs or acetaminophen for fever and pain control being the mainstay of therapy.
- To reduce the likelihood of splenic rupture, all patients should be counseled to abstain from sports until their symptoms have fully resolved.

4.4.1.5 Epiglottitis

- Epiglottitis was once predominantly a disease of children caused primarily by *Haemophilus influenzae* type b.
- Due to immunizations, a shift in the responsible pathogens has occurred, with *Staphylococcus aureus*, *Streptococcus pneumoniae*, *Streptococcus pyogenes*, and anaerobes now commonly implicated.
- Along with this, the burden of disease has shifted primarily to adults.
- Classically, pediatric patients presented with a triad of drooling, stridor, and tripod positioning, a presentation that has become much less common with the epidemiologic shift.
- Recent case series have demonstrated that painful or difficult swallowing and voice changes are the most common presenting symptoms [4].
- Fortunately, as a consequence of adult patients' larger airways, the need for airway protection in those with epiglottitis has decreased.
- Patients with respiratory distress or stridor associated with a presumed or confirmed diagnosis should be intubated, preferably in an operative room setting or by awake fiber-optic intubation.
- Clinicians should remain vigilant regarding the need for potential airway intervention in others, particularly those with:
  - Reported dyspnea
  - Rapid onset of symptoms
  - Tachycardia
  - Tachypnea [4]
- Diagnosis can be confirmed by lateral soft tissue X-rays showing an enlarged epiglottis ("thumbprint sign") or CT.
- If such imaging is pursued, it must be done in a closely supervised manner.
- Early otolaryngological consultation and empiric antibiotics should be initiated.
- Typical regimens include ampicillin/sulbactam or a third-generation cephalosporin (such as ceftriaxone) with vancomycin.

4.4.1.6 Peritonsillar Abscess

- Tonsillitis and other oropharyngeal infections can occasionally progress to abscess formation posterior to the tonsil.
- Patients present with sore throat and fever and may also have voice changes, trismus, and drooling.
- On exam, inferomedial displacement of the affected tonsil results in uvular deviation away from the abscess.
- Group A streptococci are the most frequent cause; however, many infections are polymicrobial, with anaerobes frequently identified in cultured aspirates.
- If the diagnosis is unclear after physical exam, CT and ultrasound (in the hands of an experienced operator) have been shown to have excellent sensitivity and specificity for the diagnosis.
- Ultrasound can also be useful in assisting drainage at the bedside.
- Treatment consists of drainage (typically by needle aspiration), antibiotics, and pain control.
- Typically, antibiotic regimens include amoxicillin/clavulanate 875 mg bid or clindamycin 300 mg four times daily.
  - The role of steroids is controversial.
- Admission is appropriate for patients that:
  - Cannot tolerate oral intake.
  - Have intractable pain.
  - Have immunocompromising conditions.
  - There is concern for ability to maintain their airway [1, 5, 6].

4.4.1.7 Retropharyngeal Abscess

- Retropharyngeal abscesses are most common in children under 5 years old.
- Adult patients typically have a history of an immunocompromising conditions or have recently undergone surgery or experienced trauma to the oropharynx.
- Symptoms range from fever and neck pain to neck stiffness, a "hot potato voice," and respiratory difficulty.
- The symptoms are generally quite nonspecific—and unfortunately can be rapidly progressive—therefore, a high index of suspicion is warranted.
- CT is the diagnostic test of choice.
- Infection is typically polymicrobial, including anaerobic bacteria.
- Treatment includes airway protection as needed, IV antibiotics (ampicillin/sulbactam or clindamycin, with vancomycin added if concern for MRSA), and early surgical consultation for consideration of drainage.
- Delay in diagnosis can lead to extension to contiguous structures, resulting in airway obstruction, sepsis, mediastinitis, and neurologic sequelae.

4.4.1.8 Diphtheria

- As a result of vaccination, diphtheria is exceedingly rare in the developed world.
- However, it is important to consider this disease in unvaccinated patients from underdeveloped nations.

- Symptoms are similar to many more benign viral illnesses, including gradual onset of sore throat, low-grade fever, malaise, and lymphadenopathy.
- The presence of an adherent gray pseudomembrane in the throat is pathognomonic but not universally present.
- Treatment includes airway protection, diphtheria antitoxin, and penicillin.

4.4.1.9 Salivary Gland Disease

- Three paired sets of glands (parotid, submandibular, and sublingual) are largely responsible for saliva production.
- The parotid gland is drained by Stensen's duct, while Wharton's duct drains the submandibular gland, as well as some of the secretions of the sublingual gland.
- Salivary duct stones (sialolithiasis) most frequently occur in Wharton's duct.
- Patients present with abrupt onset of pain, typically exacerbated by eating.
- Swelling of the associated gland is also commonly noted.
- Presence of purulent drainage signifies a concomitant bacterial infection. A palpable or visible stone may be present, making the diagnosis obvious. In other cases, imaging with CT or ultrasound is necessary to clarify the diagnosis. Management includes massage/milking of the affected gland and duct, analgesia, and use of sialogogues such as hard candy and acidic juice. Prompt otolaryngology follow-up is also indicated [7].
- Inflammation of a salivary duct is termed sialoadenitis.

4.4.1.10 Parotitis

- The parotid gland is most commonly affected, and the resulting process is referred to as parotitis.
- Bacterial parotitis is most commonly due to *S. aureus*, although polymicrobial infection also involving *Streptococcus viridans* and anaerobes is not unusual.
- Dehydration is a very common predisposing factor.
- Patients typically present with painful unilateral swelling of the cheek.
- Fever is common, and patients may appear quite ill. Bilateral involvement can occur in up to 25% of patients.
- Purulent drainage from Wharton's duct clinches the diagnosis.
- In other patients, ultrasonography or CT can be considered.
  - These modalities can also assess for the presence of any abscess or stone.
- Treatment includes antibiotics with coverage of *S. aureus* and anaerobes.
- Patients with toxic appearance, significant comorbidities, and poor access to otolaryngology follow-up should be admitted.
- Others can be discharged with close follow-up and an oral agent such as clindamycin.
- Amoxicillin/clavulanate may be employed if methicillin-resistant *S. aureus* is not a particular concern.
- All patients should receive hydration, analgesia, sialogogues, and parotid massage.

- Any medications that could be contributing to salivary stasis (e.g., anticholinergics) should be discontinued if possible.
- Viral parotitis is commonly associated with mumps, but influenza, parainfluenza, and other viral pathogens are also responsible.
- In contrast to bacterial parotitis, patients typically present with bilateral parotid pain and swelling which develops following a several-day period of influenza-like symptoms.
- The presence of facial erythema or warmth, or purulent drainage from Stensen's duct, is consistent with a bacterial, rather than viral, etiology.
- Treatment of viral parotitis is largely supportive and consists of analgesics and hydration.
- If there is any uncertainty as to whether the patient may have a bacterial etiology, antibiotics should be considered [5–7].

4.4.1.11 Dental Issues

Minor Dental Trauma

- The Ellis classification is used to describe the depth of a dental fracture.
- Ellis I fractures involve only the enamel and will not produce pain.
  - Patients can be referred to a dentist for further care if appearance is a concern.
- Ellis II fractures involve the enamel and the yellow dentin.
  - Pain may be present.
  - Treatment consists of analgesia and application of calcium hydroxide paste over the affected area.
  - Patients should be referred to a dentist promptly and advised to avoid any trauma to the area (including chewing), until evaluated by a dentist.
- Ellis III fractures involve the enamel, dentin, and pulp and are tooth threatening.
  - The presence of a red area in the affected tooth is the hallmark of diagnosis.
  - Patients typically report severe pain.
  - Calcium hydroxide should be applied, and the patient is referred to a dentist within 48 h.
- Avulsed permanent teeth should be re-implanted as soon as possible as the likelihood of healing and functionality long term is inversely proportional to time out of socket.
  - To perform this, gently rinse the tooth—*do not wipe the root*—and place into the socket taking care only to handle the tooth by the crown.
  - Stabilization of the affected tooth must then be achieved, either through a temporary splint performed in the ED or by a dentist or oral maxillofacial surgeon as soon as possible following re-implantation.
  - A soft diet is an imperative for such patients until they are cleared to advance by a dentist or oral maxillofacial surgeon [5, 6].
  - Evaluate for the possibility of an aspirated tooth with a chest X-ray in patients with a newly missing tooth that cannot be located, as a post-obstructive pneumonia can result.
  - Bronchoscopic retrieval is necessary if an aspirated tooth is identified.

Atraumatic Tooth Disease: Dental Caries and Pulpitis

- Erosion of the enamel results in the development of dental caries.
- If left untreated, the erosion may extend to the dentin and the pulp, causing pain, which is typically worsened by heat or cold.
- This erosion also enables invasion of bacteria from the oropharynx.
- Inflammation of the pulp resulting from this process is termed pulpitis and can be divided into reversible (acute) and irreversible (chronic) forms.
- Reversible pulpitis is typically associated with brief episodes of pain, while the pain of irreversible pulpitis is typically much longer in duration (although it tends to be less severe).
- All patients should be provided adequate analgesia, including the offering of local anesthesia with a long-acting agent such as bupivacaine.
- NSAIDs and acetaminophen are first-line therapy for dental pain.
- If refractory, brief, sparing courses of opiates may be considered.
- Systemic antibiotics are often prescribed and should be prescribed if clear evidence of infection is present (e.g., an abscess as described below) [5–7].
  - Otherwise, the utility of antibiotics is unclear [8].
- If utilized, antibiotics should cover *Streptococcus mutans* and other oral anaerobes.
  - Penicillin VK 500 mg four times daily or amoxicillin 500 mg four times daily are appropriate first-line choices (clindamycin or erythromycin may be used in penicillin-allergic patients).
- Prompt dental referral is appropriate for all patients with pulpitis. Definitive treatment of irreversible pulpitis is either extraction or root canal therapy.

Periapical Abscess

- If pulpitis is left untreated, bacteria may invade the alveolar bone and contiguous tissues, forming a periapical abscess.
- Patients may present with pain, swelling, or complaint of drainage of pus (with its associated foul taste).
- Treatment includes immediate incision and drainage, irrigation, and antibiotics as described above.
- Patients should be referred to a dentist for root canal therapy or extraction.

Ludwig's Angina

- Ludwig's angina, cellulitis of the submandibular space, may result if the above processes occur in the region of the second and third molar, allowing bacterial invasion of the submandibular space (extension of deep space infections of the oropharynx can also cause Ludwig's angina).
- Patients typically present with pain, edema, and a hoarse voice.
- Submandibular swelling, which can precipitously progress to tongue elevation resulting in airway occlusion, is noted on exam.

- Initial management includes immediate airway assessment and securing of a definitive airway if indicated.
- Close re-evaluation is imperative in patients without an established definitive airway.
- Prompt oral maxillofacial surgery consultation is necessary, as is administration of parenteral antibiotics to cover the typical polymicrobial infection.
  - Ampicillin/sulbactam and clindamycin are appropriate choices [5–7].

4.4.1.12 Periodontal Disease

Gingivitis

- Gingivitis, inflammation of the gingiva, is a reversible inflammatory response to irritants including plaque.
- Edema, erythema, and occasional bleeding or discharge may be present.
- Patients should be referred to a dentist for debridement.
- In the interim, patients should be counseled on the role of improved oral hygiene.

Periodontitis

- If untreated, gingivitis can progress to periodontitis, an irreversible inflammatory condition that can result in destruction of the periodontal ligament and alveolar bone.
- As a result, patients may present with loosened/lost teeth.
- Prompt referral to a dentist is indicated.

Periodontal Abscesses

- With progression of periodontitis, an abscess may form in the areas of eroded gum and alveolar bone tissue; such abscesses are termed periodontal abscesses and differ from periapical abscesses in that the adjacent tooth may be otherwise healthy.
- Incision and drainage as well as irrigation of such abscesses should be performed at the time of diagnosis.
- Patients are typically prescribed a short course of antibiotics active against typical oral flora, as described above.
- All patients should be referred promptly for dental follow-up for consideration of further debridement of tissue, as well as provided with adequate analgesia.

Necrotizing Ulcerative Gingivitis

- Necrotizing ulcerative gingivitis (Vincent's disease, trench mouth) refers to a direct bacterial invasion of gingival tissue, rather than the simple inflammation characteristic of gingivitis.
- Risk factors include:
  - Malnutrition.
  - Smoking.

  - Emotional stress.
  - Immunocompromised status (particularly HIV).
  - Poor hygiene.
- Patients commonly present with rapid onset of pain, as well as foul-smelling breath and a metallic taste, and may also have associated fever and lymphadenopathy.
- On exam, edematous interdental gingival papillae with ulceration and bleeding are noted.
- A friable pseudomembrane may also be present.
- Treatment consists of improved oral hygiene, antiseptic mouthwash (e.g., 3% hydrogen peroxide, chlorhexidine), systemic analgesics, and topical anesthetics (e.g., viscous lidocaine).
- If systemic symptoms are present, oral antibiotics should also be prescribed.
- Patients should be referred to a dentist for further care [5–7].

Pericoronitis

- Inflammation of the gingival tissue overlying an impacted tooth crown (typically the third molar) is termed pericoronitis.
- Due to proximity to vital structures, left untreated, the condition has the potential to become life-threatening.
- Pain is often severe and is worsened by chewing and mouth opening.
- Trismus may be present. Warm saline irrigation, rinses with antiseptic mouthwash, and analgesics should be provided.
- If symptoms are severe, or there are signs of systemic illness, antibiotics should be provided.
- If an abscess is present, careful incision and drainage should be performed.
- Patients should be referred to an oral maxillofacial surgeon for extraction of the offending molar.

4.4.1.13 Post-extraction Pain

- Pain in the immediate 1–2 days following dental extraction is common and ideally treated with systemic analgesics such as acetaminophen, NSAIDs, or opiates, as well as application of ice packs.
  - An opioid may be considered for breakthrough pain.
- Alveolar osteitis, commonly referred to as dry socket, typically develops 3–4 days post-extraction if the blood clot at the site of the extraction is displaced.
- A localized infection may occur at the site.
  - Pain is typically abrupt in onset and quite severe.
- Following local anesthesia, management typically consists of gentle irrigation followed by packing of the site with gauze soaked in eugenol or one of several commercially available dressings designed for this indication.
- Patients should be discharged with oral analgesics and follow up with their dentist within 24 h.
- Antibiotics active against oral flora are also typically provided.

References

1. Cirilli AR. Emergency evaluation and management of the sore throat. Emerg Med Clin N Am. 2013;31:501–15.
2. Wessels MR. Clinical practice: streptococcal pharyngitis, vol. 364. N Engl J Med; 2011. p. 648–55.
3. Son KH, Shin MY. Clinical features of Epstein-Barr virus-associated infectious mononucleosis in hospitalized Korean children. Korean J Pediatr. 2011;54:409–13.
4. Guardiani E, Bliss M, Harley E. Supraglottitis in the era following widespread immunization against *Haemophilus influenzae* type B: evolving principles in diagnosis and management. Laryngoscope. 2010;120:2183–8.
5. Marx JA, Hockberger RS, Walls RM. Rosen's emergency medicine—concepts and clinical practice. 8th ed. Philadelphia: Elsevier Saunders; 2013.
6. Tintinalli JE, Stapczynski J, Ma O, Yealy DM, Meckler GD, Cline DM, editors. Tintinalli's emergency medicine: a comprehensive study guide. 8th ed. New York: McGraw-Hill; 2016.
7. Armstrong MA. Salivary gland emergencies. Emerg Med Clin N Am. 2013;31:481–99.
8. Hodgdon A. Dental and related infections. Emerg Med Clin N Am. 2013;31:465–80.

Demystifying the Enigma of the Pediatric Viral Upper Respiratory Infection

5

Harman Kaur and Sakina Sojar

5.1 Introduction

Viral upper respiratory infections (URIs) are typically acute, self-limiting illnesses that can present with cough, congestion, rhinorrhea, fevers, otitis media, headaches, and generalized malaise. Common viruses include rhinovirus, adenovirus, influenza, enterovirus, respiratory syncytial virus (RSV), and coronavirus [1]. While rhinovirus is present for most of the year, adenovirus, RSV, and coronavirus are predominantly present throughout the winter [2], though these patterns are changing in light of the present COVID-19 pandemic [3]. Enterovirus is most often present in summer, and parainfluenza in late fall. Children younger than 6 years of age can have as many as six to eight viral URIs per year [4]. In 2011, 28% of pediatric emergency department (ED) visits were for infectious disease-related causes, 41% of those being for viral URIs [5].

5.2 Presentation

Patients will typically present with cough, congestion, rhinorrhea, and fevers. Fever is usually present in the first few days and first to resolve. Cough is typically the most bothersome symptom and is usually the reason for presentation to the ED. Even

H. Kaur
Division of Pediatric Emergency Medicine, Arnold Palmer Hospital For Children, Orlando, FL, USA

S. Sojar (✉)
Division of Pediatric Emergency Medicine, Warren Alpert Medical School of Brown University, Providence, RI, USA
e-mail: sakina.sojar@brownphysicians.org

B. K. Desai et al. (eds.), *Primary Care for Emergency Physicians*,
https://doi.org/10.1007/978-3-031-64676-8_5

after resolution of other symptoms, cough can persist for 1–2 weeks. Other associated symptoms include difficulty feeding in infants, decreased appetite in children, increasing fussiness, and difficulty sleeping. Sometimes, viral URIs are also associated with emesis or diarrhea. Emesis is often described as post-tussive, triggered after bouts of forceful coughing. Symptoms of viral URIs will usually peak at about days 2–3 but can last up to 14 days after onset [6].

5.3 Diagnostic Workup

Diagnosis is made clinically based on symptoms, exposures, and physical exam. The physician should consider broadening the differential to include more than viral URIs if patient's temperature is greater than 39 °C and if the patient is ill appearing and has adventitious sounds on lung exam, hemoptysis, or difficulty breathing. Without focal findings on auscultation of the lungs, a chest X-ray is not indicated. A respiratory viral panel can be performed to identify the viral etiology but will not typically change management aside from verifying the source of symptoms or isolation guidelines.

If a fever recurs shortly after resolution of a suspected viral illness, or if the fever lasts for greater than 5 days, the patient may warrant evaluation for secondary bacterial infections such as acute otitis media (AOM), pneumonia, and sinusitis, inflammatory syndromes such as Kawasaki disease, multisystem inflammatory syndrome in children, malignancy, or rheumatologic disease.

5.4 Special Considerations in Pediatric Viral URI

5.4.1 Acute Otitis Media

Acute otitis media (AOM) is a complication of acute viral URI in pediatric patients due to Eustachian tube dysfunction related to shorter and more horizontal positioning compared to adults. AOM should be considered in children with moderate to severe bulging of the tympanic membrane and new-onset otorrhea and in those with mild bulging of the tympanic membrane with recent onset of ear pain or intense erythema with loss of light reflex of the tympanic membrane [7]. AOM should not be diagnosed in children who do not have middle ear effusion [7].

5.4.2 Conjunctivitis

A viral URI can be accompanied by conjunctivitis. Patients will typically report that the child woke up with his or her eyes crusted shut and that they have then had clear drainage with eye redness. Viral conjunctivitis is transmitted by direct contact with infected secretions especially in clinic settings where an infected patient has likely touched multiple surfaces [8].

Certain symptoms at presentation may be more indicative of bacterial conjunctivitis and should be treated appropriately. In a meta-analysis review by Johnson et al. it was demonstrated that associated symptoms of pharyngitis and enlarged preauricular nodes with history of contact with another person with conjunctival injection were more indicative of viral conjunctivitis, while the presence of mucopurulent discharge and otitis media was more indicative of bacterial conjunctivitis [9].

5.4.3 Croup

Laryngotracheobronchitis, more commonly known as croup, is a complication of acute viral infection. It is known to be caused by parainfluenza virus, though several viruses can cause this condition. Croup presents as a barking cough with inspiratory stridor and hoarseness as a result of inflammation in the larynx and subglottic airway. More severe disease can cause narrowing of the airway which can cause visible respiratory distress [10]. More recently, SARS-CoV-2 infection that has caused croup in pediatric patients has required more aggressive intervention than typical management of croup caused by parainfluenza [11].

5.4.4 Sinusitis

Sinusitis is less likely in younger children given that the sinuses are not completely developed. The maxillary sinuses are present at birth and go through rapid expansion by age 4 years, and the sphenoid sinuses begin to develop during the first 2 years of life. The paranasal sinuses reach near adult proportions by age 12 years [12]. Sinusitis should be considered in the appropriate age group if congestion persists for greater than 10 days, purulent nasal discharge is present for 3–4 days, there is new onset/recurrence of fever, or temperature is greater than 39 °C [13].

5.5 Management

Before discussing management of a viral URI, it is important to remember if the patient is less than 2 months of age and presenting with a fever, a neonatal sepsis workup should be considered.

Primary prevention of viral URIs is through frequent handwashing and avoiding touching one's face.

Management is predominantly supportive.

- *Congestion*
  - Nasal saline spray to break up mucus with frequent suctioning with either bulb suction or devices such as a manual nasal aspirator.
  - Creating a steamy environment in the bathroom/shower where the child can sit supervised for 20–30 min at a time.

  - Humidifiers in the room where the child sleeps to thin secretions.
  - If pursuing nasal irrigation, it is important to emphasize the use of sterile or bottled water instead of tap water due to the risk of amebic encephalitis with tap water [14].
  - Discourage oxymetazoline use for congestion due to rebound congestion.
- *Cough/sore throat*
  - Honey or honey-containing tea with lemon for sore throat or cough, specifically at night to help with sleep. Honey is not recommended for children younger than 12 months. In patients <12 months of age, agave may be a suitable alternative.
  - In patients with a history of reactive airway disease or asthma, albuterol as needed for cough for the first few days of illness can prevent exacerbation.
  - The AAP advises against the use of codeine- and dextromethorphan-containing cough products in children [15].
  - The FDA does not recommend cough and cold medications for children younger than 2 years of age [16].
- *Fever*
  - Fevers, or a temperature >38 °C, can be treated with appropriate weight-based doses of acetaminophen and ibuprofen. Ibuprofen is not recommended for children under the age of 6 months.
  - Aspirin should be avoided in children with viral URIs due to the risk of Reye syndrome.
- *Vomiting/diarrhea*
  - Adequate hydration is essential. One can supplement with oral rehydration solutions such as Pedialyte in infants who cannot tolerate formula/breast milk or have decreased appetite or increased losses through vomiting or diarrhea.
  - Some children may require a prescription for ondansetron to help treat vomiting and allow for oral rehydration.
- *Acute Otitis Media (AOM)*
  - As many as 50% of viral URIs are unnecessarily treated with antibiotics, and in children, acute otitis media is often the reason that antibiotics are prescribed [17]. Multiple studies have demonstrated that antibiotic therapy for acute otitis media serves limited benefit [17], and the American Academy of Pediatrics, American Academy of Family Physicians, and the European AOM guidelines support the use for watchful waiting prior to initiation of antibiotics [7].
  - Patients with non-severe symptoms can be monitored closely with outpatient follow-up and parental education. Symptoms should be monitored for progression, and antibiotics can be prescribed as warranted. Parents can be offered a prescription to fill for an antibiotic if symptoms do not resolve on their own in 2–3 days.

Watch and wait guidelines [7]
Offer observation with close follow-up for ***unilateral*** **AOM in children 6–23 months** and ***bilateral*** **AOM in children 24 months and older** without severe symptoms (mild otalgia for less than 48 h and temperature less than 39 °C)

Watch and wait guidelines [7]
If choosing observation, the child should have close follow-up, and if the child's clinical condition worsens or does not show improvement without 48–72 h of diagnosis, antibiotic therapy should be initiated
Antibiotics should be used to manage **non-severe *bilateral* AOM in children younger than 24 months** and for **severe AOM in children 6 months and older** (moderate to severe otalgia, otalgia for at least 48 h, temperature greater than 39 °C)

- Ear pain should be treated appropriately with ibuprofen and/or acetaminophen as needed.
- First-line antibiotic therapy for AOM is high-dose amoxicillin. If there is failure to respond or recurrence of AOM within 30 days, therapy should be escalated in a stepwise manner to high-dose amoxicillin-clavulanate, followed by a third-generation cephalosporin such as cefdinir or cefixime [18].
- In children with tympanostomy tubes, first-line antibiotic therapy for AOM is topical, such as ciprofloxacin or ofloxacin otic drops [19].

• *Conjunctivitis*
  - Warm or cool compress to remove crusting for symptomatic relief, antihistamine drops, or artificial tears to help with sensation of grit in the eye.
  - If it is difficult to rule out bacterial conjunctivitis, a 5–7-day course of erythromycin ointment or trimethoprim-polymyxin B ophthalmic solution can be prescribed.

• *Croup*
  - Management of croup is dependent on the severity of disease. Severity of disease can be assessed using the Westley Croup Score and clinical judgment [20].
  - Patients without stridor at rest, but with the pathognomonic barky cough, can be treated with dexamethasone as a single dose.
  - Those presenting with inspiratory stridor **at rest** should be given nebulized racemic epinephrine in addition to the single dose of dexamethasone. After an observation period in the ED, these patients may still be suitable for discharge.
  - Patients with severe stridor and respiratory distress at presentation may require several doses of nebulized racemic epinephrine, with possible escalation to heliox or intubation. Dexamethasone can be given intravenously or intramuscularly. Patients that require more than one dose of nebulized racemic epinephrine will necessitate hospital admission.
  - The tablets of dexamethasone can be crushed and dissolved as this is palatable for children compared to dexamethasone solution.

• *Sinusitis*
  - When sinusitis is a superinfection in the setting of a viral URI, *Haemophilus influenzae, Streptococcus pneumoniae, Moraxella catarrhalis,* and *Chlamydophila pneumoniae* are more likely to be the infectious organisms [21], and antibiotic therapy should be targeted toward these specific organisms.
  - Empiric treatment of sinusitis is low-dose amoxicillin-clavulanate for 10 days [13].

References

1. Pappas DE. The common cold, in principles and practice of pediatric infectious diseases. Elsevier; 2018. p. 199–202.e1.
2. Monto AS. The seasonality of rhinovirus infections and its implications for clinical recognition. Clin Ther. 2002;24(12):1987–97.
3. Groves HE, et al. The impact of the COVID-19 pandemic on influenza, respiratory syncytial virus, and other seasonal respiratory virus circulation in Canada: a population-based study. Lancet Reg Health Am. 2021;1:100015.
4. Pappas DE, Hendley JO. The common cold and decongestant therapy. Pediatr Rev. 2011;32(2):47–54. quiz 55.
5. Hasegawa K, et al. Infectious disease-related emergency department visits among children in the US. Pediatr Infect Dis J. 2015;34(7):681–5.
6. Pappas DE, et al. Symptom profile of common colds in school-aged children. Pediatr Infect Dis J. 2008;27(1):8–11.
7. Lieberthal AS, et al. The diagnosis and management of acute otitis media. Pediatrics. 2013;131(3):e964–99.
8. Azar MJ, et al. Possible consequences of shaking hands with your patients with epidemic keratoconjunctivitis. Am J Ophthalmol. 1996;121(6):711–2.
9. Johnson D, Liu D, Simel D. Does this patient with acute infectious conjunctivitis have a bacterial infection?: the rational clinical examination systematic review. JAMA. 2022;327(22):2231–7.
10. Tovar Padua LJ, Cherry JD. Croup (laryngitis, laryngotracheitis, spasmodic croup, laryngotracheobronchitis, bacterial tracheitis, and laryngotracheobronchopneumonitis) and epiglottitis (supraglottitis). In: Cherry JD, et al., editors. Feigin and Cherry's textbook of pediatric infectious diseases. Philadelphia: Elsevier; 2019. p. 175.
11. Venn AMR, Schmidt JM, Mullan PC. Pediatric croup with COVID-19. Am J Emerg Med. 2021;43:287.e1–3.
12. Wolf G, Anderhuber W, Kuhn F. Development of the paranasal sinuses in children: implications for paranasal sinus surgery. Ann Otol Rhinol Laryngol. 1993;102(9):705–11.
13. Chow AW, et al. IDSA clinical practice guideline for acute bacterial rhinosinusitis in children and adults. Clin Infect Dis. 2012;54(8):e72–e112.
14. Tap and Faucet Water. 2017. https://www.cdc.gov/parasites/naegleria/tap-faucet-water.html. Accessed 18 June 2022.
15. American Academy of Pediatrics. Committee on Drugs. Use of codeine- and dextromethorphan-containing cough remedies in children. Pediatrics. 1997;99(6):918–20.
16. Tips from the FDA to safely treat your child's cough and cold. https://www.fda.gov/consumers/consumer-updates/should-you-give-kids-medicine-coughs-and-colds. Accessed 18 June 2022.
17. Smolinski NE, Antonelli PJ, Winterstein AG. Watchful waiting for acute otitis media. Pediatrics. 2022;150(1):e2021055613.
18. Gaddey HL, Wright MT, Nelson TN. Otitis media: rapid evidence review. Am Fam Physician. 2019;100(6):350–6.
19. Rosenfeld RM, et al. Clinical practice guideline: tympanostomy tubes in children (update). Otolaryngol Head Neck Surg. 2022;166(1_suppl):S1–S55.
20. Retzke J. Croup (acute laryngotracheobronchitis). Pediatric Care Online; 2021.
21. Sawada S, Matsubara S. Microbiology of acute maxillary sinusitis in children. Laryngoscope. 2021;131(10):E2705–11.

Sinonasal Diseases

6

Graham Clifford and Charles Hwang

6.1 Allergic Rhinitis

6.1.1 Epidemiology

Allergic rhinitis (AR) is one of the most common diseases affecting both adults and children, impacting approximately one in six Americans [1, 2]. It is the most common chronic disease in children and is the fifth most common chronic disease overall in the United States [3]. Because of its prevalence, it results in a significant 6–11 billion US dollars in healthcare costs annually, as well as a 2–4 billion US dollar loss in productivity annually [1, 2, 4].

6.1.2 Pathophysiology

AR is an immunoglobulin E (IgE)-mediated disease characterized by inflammation of the lining of the nasal passages. An inciting allergen causes numerous inflammatory cells to infiltrate the nasal mucosa. T cells stimulate IgE production by plasma cells; this triggers the release of histamine and leukotrienes that cause the classic symptoms of rhinitis. These symptoms include increased mucous secretion, pruritus, rhinorrhea, nasal congestion, sneezing, postnasal drip, conjunctivitis, cough, eye itching, nasal itching, palate itching, fatigue, and sleep disturbance [4–7].

The development of AR requires sensitization to the causal allergen [8]. This typically takes a few years to develop; therefore, diagnosing AR in a child less than 2 years old is uncommon [9]. After 2 years of age, the prevalence of AR increases into early adulthood, with a decline in prevalence with older age [9–16].

G. Clifford · C. Hwang (✉)
Department of Emergency Medicine, University of Florida College of Medicine, Gainesville, FL, USA
e-mail: hwang.c@ufl.edu

B. K. Desai et al. (eds.), *Primary Care for Emergency Physicians*,
https://doi.org/10.1007/978-3-031-64676-8_6

Another interesting feature of AR is its seemingly higher prevalence in the industrialized and urban areas of the world over the past century. Some theories suggest the observed increase in prevalence of AR is due to the urban hypothesis (e.g., increased hygiene, decline in parasitic infections, lifestyle changes, decrease in environmental toxins) [17–20]. Ultimately, the factors that lead to the development of AR are vast as well as complex, and there is likely no one singular cause for this observed increase in prevalence. More high-quality studies are needed to draw definitive conclusions on the matter.

6.1.3 Diagnosis

The diagnosis of AR is based on history and physical examination. Frequently, AR goes undetected because patients do not realize the impact AR has on quality of life, nor do providers regularly screen patients for its signs and symptoms [6]. Symptoms suggestive of AR include nasal itching, nasal congestion, sniffling, rhinorrhea, sneezing, and conjunctivitis triggered by an allergic cause. These triggers may include dust mites, pollen, animal dander, upholstery, cockroach residues, mold, and humidity. Perennial symptoms are more suggestive of indoor allergens such as dust mites and animal dander, while seasonal symptoms are more suggestive of outdoor allergens. It should be noted that outdoor allergens may cause perennial symptoms in more temperate climates. The timeline for development of these symptoms is closely correlated with histamine concentration [21, 22]. Following allergen exposure, an immediate response is expected secondary to mast cell degranulation; these symptoms typically peak at 15–30 min after that exposure with a return to baseline after approximately 1 h [21–23]. A late-phase reaction develops in around 50% of patients with seasonal AR. Late-onset maximal symptoms have been observed to peak at 6–12 h after allergen exposure and are thought to be secondary to both mast cell degranulation and basophil influx [22–25]. Atypical symptoms, such as unilateral nasal symptoms, severe headache, epistaxis, or anosmia, may suggest a more insidious diagnosis (e.g., CSF rhinorrhea, chronic rhinosinusitis, sinonasal tumor, and granulomatous disease) [4, 26]. Other sinonasal pathologies, such as sinusitis, granulomatous disease, and viral upper respiratory infections, can cause symptoms similar to AR and should be further delineated [4].

The World Health Organization in 2001 assisted in the development of a classification system defining AR by its pattern of symptoms. First, they classified AR temporally using the verbiage "intermittent," meaning less than 4 days per week or less than 4 weeks per year. Second, they classified AR using the verbiage "persistent," meaning greater than 4 days per week or greater than 4 weeks per year. Third, they quantified AR by the severity of the symptoms (mild or moderate severe) [6, 27]. The severity is classified based on the impact on quality of life; mild severity indicates symptoms that do not interfere with quality of life, whereas moderate severe symptoms do [28]. In contrast, the United States Food and Drug Administration prefers to classify AR as "seasonal," meaning symptoms occurring at a certain time of year, or "perennial," meaning symptoms occurring year-round. Although these categories separate AR into rigid compartments. AR is an inflammatory disease that exists on a continuum. For example, patients living in more temperate climates may experience significant overlap between seasonal and perennial symptoms. Moreover, patients with perennial AR may have seasonal exacerbations based on local temperature and climate changes. Furthermore, many experts consider AR on a spectrum of diseases that includes the entire respiratory tract, including asthma and reactive airway disease [6, 27]. However, these classifications of AR help guide the clinician toward the appropriate treatment for each patient [4].

The patient may have a past medical history or family history of asthma, sleep apnea, sinusitis, otitis media, nasal polyps, atopic dermatitis, or conjunctivitis [4, 6, 29, 30]. Many commonly prescribed medications may cause nasal symptoms and should be elicited as well; these include antihypertensives, acetylsalicylic acid, non-steroidal anti-inflammatory drugs, psychotropic medications, topical decongestants, and recreational misadventures [4, 6, 31].

The physical examination may include clear rhinorrhea, nasal congestion, pale discoloration of the nasal mucosa, postnasal drip, and lacrimation. Conjunctival edema, as well as the classic "allergic shiner," or periorbital darkness and puffiness, may be present. Patients may be observed to have sequelae or behavioral adaptations due to long-standing AR, including mouth breathing, frequent sniffling, throat clearing, or the development of an "allergic crease" from frequent rubbing of the nose. This "allergic crease" is also known as the "allergic salute." The physical examination should evaluate for other insidious causes of nasal obstruction and rhinorrhea, including CSF leak, nasal polyps, or foreign bodies [4, 6].

Although the definitive diagnosis of AR is by IgE testing and identification of a specific allergen that causes symptoms, it is reasonable to make a clinical diagnosis based on the history and physical exam and to initiate empiric therapy. This is reasonable especially if the symptoms are adversely impacting quality of life. Routine laboratory testing will usually be normal; neither eosinophil counts nor total serum IgE levels are sensitive enough alone to rule out AR [32]. Providers should make the provisional diagnosis of AR when patients present with symptoms of AR and the history and physical examination are suggestive of an allergic cause [4]. Moreover, symptomatic improvement from allergen avoidance and/or empiric therapy further supports the diagnosis of AR and may preclude further allergy testing altogether [4]. It is worth noting that a positive response to glucocorticoids and antihistamines does not establish a definitive diagnosis of AR as these therapies can also be effective in the treatment of nonallergic rhinitis [32, 33]. Routine imaging does not play a role in the diagnosis of uncomplicated AR; it exposes patients to excessive cost and the risk of ionizing radiation without any benefits in diagnosis. However, if there is clinical concern for other pathology, including neoplasm, abscess, or rhinosinusitis, imaging may be indicated [34].

6.1.4 Management

In the treatment of AR, empiric therapy for allergic rhinitis includes avoidance of triggers, environmental modification, and medical management. Clinicians may advise patients to avoid known allergen triggers and recommend low-cost, potentially beneficial lifestyle modifications that reduce the allergen burden within the environment. This includes removal of pets, installation of air purification systems, and the use of bed covers. Numerous studies have evaluated pet ownership, dander elimination by frequent pet washing, the use of impermeable bed covers, air filtration using high-efficacy particulate air (HEPA) filters, and acaricides (chemical agents to kill dust mites). Although these interventions reduce allergen levels, no single intervention has been proven to be effective for AR, and a multiple intervention strategy may prove useful; further studies need to be performed [4, 35–39].

Intranasal steroids are considered the most effective medication in treating AR and are more effective than oral antihistamines [40–46]. Intranasal steroids include mometasone, beclomethasone, budesonide, fluticasone, and triamcinolone. Short courses of systemic glucocorticoids may be indicated for severe AR that is affecting a patient's quality of life drastically (i.e., work and sleep disturbances) but should not be given repeatedly or for prolonged periods of time [47].

Patients with intermittent symptoms may be treated with second-generation, nonsedating antihistamines and/or decongestants. The second-generation antihistamines include cetirizine, fexofenadine, loratadine, levocetirizine, and desloratadine and are efficacious in decreasing symptoms of AR but are not as efficacious as inhaled glucocorticoids. For example, antihistamines have poorer performance in improving nasal congestion [42, 48]. Intranasal antihistamines, such as azelastine, are also effective at managing AR symptoms while minimizing systemic side effects [42, 49].

Patients with refractory AR should be referred to a specialist for possible immunotherapy. Special consideration should be taken when treating AR in young children less than 2 years old, pregnant patients, and lactating patients.

Clinicians should refer patients for IgE allergy testing when the diagnosis is uncertain, when patients do not respond to empiric therapy, or when identification of the specific allergen will help guide therapy [4]. IgE allergy testing is performed either by skin or blood testing. Skin testing is a highly sensitive and specific test that allows direct observation of the body's response to a suspected allergen after introducing the allergen intradermally (either by skin pricking or by intradermal injection) [50, 51]. Blood testing is performed by an immunoassay; allergen-specific IgE is incubated with the suspected allergen, which has been attached to a solid phase. The bound IgE complex is then measured by introducing anti-IgE antibody (specific for the allergen) that has been radioactively or enzymatically labeled [4]. There are other tests that are used to evaluate suspected AR, including acoustic rhinometry, olfactory testing, microarray testing, nasal allergen challenges, and nasal eosinophilia smears although there is presently insufficient evidence on their utility [4].

6.2 Sinusitis

6.2.1 Epidemiology

Sinusitis affects approximately one in eight American adults, or 35 million American adults, per year [52, 53]. More than 20% of prescribed antibiotics are for sinusitis, making sinusitis the fifth most common diagnosis treated with antibiotics [54, 55]. The healthcare-related costs associated with managing sinusitis exceed $11 billion per year, in addition to losses in productivity and quality of life [53, 56]. Despite the prevalence of sinusitis, significant variations exist in its management [57]. Moreover, sinusitis is not a benign disease; besides the prevalence and financial impact of sinusitis, uncommon but serious complications can include meningitis, intracerebral abscess, orbital cellulitis, and orbital abscess [58].

6.2.2 Pathophysiology

Acute sinusitis is commonly caused by viral infections. The most common viral causes include rhinovirus, influenza virus, and parainfluenza virus. Inoculation by viruses occurs via direct contact with the nasal mucosa. These viruses can spread to the paranasal sinuses by direct spread. Another method of spread interestingly occurs when a patient blows one's nose, elevating intranasal pressures and propelling the virus into the paranasal sinuses. The subsequent inflammation, vascular permeability, hypersecretion, and impaired ciliary clearance result in sinus obstruction and the classic syndrome of sinusitis [59]. Because this inflammation typically also involves the contiguous nasal passages as well, many experts prefer the more correct term *rhinosinusitis*. Although viruses are the most common cause of acute rhinosinusitis, any inflammatory cause that obstructs the sinonasal passages can cause acute rhinosinusitis (ARS), including allergic rhinitis, nasal obstruction or polyps, dental infection, and impaired mucociliary clearance [60]. ARS can become secondarily infected by bacteria and occurs in 0.5–2% of patients with ARS [57, 59, 61]. Common bacteria associated with bacterial sinusitis are *Streptococcus pneumoniae*, *Haemophilus influenzae*, and *Moraxella catarrhalis*.

6.2.3 Diagnosis

Rhinosinusitis is categorized by the duration of symptoms and by the etiology. ARS refers to symptoms lasting shorter than 4 weeks, while chronic rhinosinusitis refers to symptoms that persist more than 12 weeks [57]. ARS is further categorized by its etiology, bacterial versus viral. This distinction is important, as antibiotics are not indicated for viral causes. Bacterial sinusitis is further classified by its clinical manifestations, complicated versus uncomplicated; these are distinguished by whether there is clinical evidence of extension outside of the paranasal sinuses and nasal cavity. Four or more discrete episodes of sinusitis in a year are termed recurrent rhinosinusitis. Expert opinion varies on the terminology for symptoms that last between 4 and 12 weeks, with some experts labeling this ARS and others labeling this subacute. Therefore, the management of symptoms lasting from 4 to 12 weeks must be tailored to the individual patient [57].

Symptoms suggestive of rhinosinusitis include nasal congestion, rhinorrhea, postnasal drip, purulent (not clear) nasal discharge, teeth discomfort, facial pain localized over the frontal or maxillary sinuses, facial pressure or fullness, fever, fatigue, cough, malaise, anosmia, headache, and ear pressure/fullness. Symptoms may worsen with straining or bending over [57, 62–65].

Clinical findings of rhinosinusitis include nasal discharge, rhinorrhea, purulent drainage from the nose or oropharynx, mucosal edema, or turbinate hyperemia or hypertrophy. Patients may exhibit alteration in speech tone secondary to nasal obstruction. The affected sinus may have overlying erythema, edema, or tenderness to palpation and percussion. The maxillary teeth may exhibit tenderness to percussion if the maxillary sinus is involved. Transillumination of the sinuses may show opacification of the frontal and/or maxillary sinuses although this is neither sensitive nor specific [57, 64, 66]. Of these physical findings, purulence within the nasal cavity is the only finding shown to have diagnostic value [57]. The provider should also evaluate for complications of sinusitis, including nuchal rigidity, abnormal extraocular movements and diplopia, altered mental status, visual changes, facial or preseptal or orbital cellulitis, and proptosis [57].

The diagnosis of ARS is a clinical diagnosis; the diagnosis is made when a patient has up to 4 weeks of purulent nasal discharge associated with nasal obstruction and/or facial pain or pressure. Distinguishing between viral and bacterial rhinosinusitis is trickier, as the symptoms of acute viral (nonbacterial) rhinosinusitis have significant overlap with that of acute bacterial rhinosinusitis [57].

The clinical course of acute viral rhinosinusitis is similar to other viral upper respiratory tract infections (URIs); patients typically are afebrile but may have a fever early on that precedes the onset of self-limited respiratory symptoms. Once the fever abates early in the disease course, respiratory symptoms usually peak in severity between days 3 and 6 of illness and should continue to improve by day 10 of illness [64].

On the contrary, symptoms of acute bacterial rhinosinusitis typically last longer than 10 days, and symptoms are generally more severe. The American Academy of Otolaryngology Clinical Practice Guideline provides criteria to assist in making a diagnosis of acute bacterial rhinosinusitis. First, the guideline states that when a patient has persistent symptoms of ARS without clinical improvement for 10 days, the diagnosis of acute bacterial rhinosinusitis can be made. The second criteria state that if a patient exhibits symptoms of ARS that initially improve but then worsen, with a total course of illness greater than or equal to 10 days, a diagnosis of acute bacterial rhinosinusitis can be made [57, 67]. It is important to note that the presence or absence of purulent drainage does not distinguish viral from bacterial infections [68]. Moreover, the Clinical Practice Guideline does not include fever as a distinguishing factor between viral and bacterial rhinosinusitis, as fever may be present in patients with viral rhinosinusitis. Fever has a sensitivity and specificity of approximately 50% for bacterial rhinosinusitis [69, 70]. Certain experts, however, encourage careful consideration of acute bacterial rhinosinusitis in the subgroup of patients with "high fever" and purulent nasal discharge for 3–4 days. The Infectious Diseases Society of America defines "high fever" as greater than 39 °C [63, 64, 67].

It is difficult for radiographic imaging to distinguish bacterial from viral rhinosinusitis unless features of complicated bacterial rhinosinusitis are evident (i.e., spread beyond the nasal cavity and paranasal sinuses). For routine acute rhinosinusitis, radiographic imaging is not indicated unless a complication or alternative diagnosis is suspected [57, 64]. Complications of sinusitis include orbital or intracranial extension, such as preseptal cellulitis, orbital cellulitis, subperiosteal abscess, meningitis, intracranial or epidural abscess, osteomyelitis, or cavernous sinus thrombosis [71]. Alternative diagnoses such as malignancy or granulomatous disease may warrant imaging as well.

Clinicians should also have a heightened level of suspicion in patients with an immunocompromised state or diabetes which predisposes patients to complications. Of particular concern for immunocompromised patients or patients with diabetes is invasive fungal rhinosinusitis, typically caused by aspergillosis, mucormycosis, and dematiaceous molds [72, 73]. Survival can be poor [74]. Therefore, imaging with CT or MRI should be performed when invasive fungal rhinosinusitis is suspected, and biopsy is needed to assist in guidance of therapy [75, 76].

6.2.4 Management

In viral rhinosinusitis, viruses cause a marked inflammatory response mediated by cytokines, resulting in mucosal edema, mucus production, and impaired ciliary function. Antibiotics are not effective for viral illnesses; rather, the management should be directed at symptomatic relief. Palliative medications directed toward symptom control, such as antipyretics, analgesics, nonsteroidal anti-inflammatory drugs, nasal saline irrigation, decongestants, antihistamines, antitussives, and topical corticosteroids, may drastically improve symptomatic relief [77, 78].

For bacterial rhinosinusitis, symptomatic management (as discussed above) may prove useful because pain relief is often a principal reason patients seek healthcare. A meta-analysis was conducted on the use of inhaled glucocorticoids as an adjunct to antibiotic therapy in the treatment of acute bacterial rhinosinusitis and found a number needed to treat of 15 patients treated with inhaled glucocorticoids to improve the clinical outcome for one patient [67]. Given the low side effect profile of inhaled glucocorticoids, it is worth clinical consideration when treating acute bacterial rhinosinusitis. With respect to antibiotic therapy, when comparing placebo versus antibiotic therapy, the evidence remains equivocal with respect to cure rate, duration of illness, and adverse events [57]. Therefore, clinicians may offer watchful waiting or antibiotic therapy, both of which are appropriate, evidence-based practices. Watchful waiting refers to symptomatic management while deferring antibiotics for 7 days. Antibiotics are started if symptoms do not improve after

7 days or worsen at any time. Special consideration should be given to immunocompromised patients as watchful waiting could be potentially harmful in this patient subset; there is a paucity of meaningful evidence to provide further guidance. Watchful waiting, along with anticipatory guidance and return precautions, should only be offered if follow-up is guaranteed to ensure that antibiotics may be started in a timely manner [57, 64]. Patients concerned about healthcare access may also be offered a safety net antibiotic prescription, which can be filled after a period of watchful waiting. Joint decision-making between the clinician and patient, including the risks, benefits, and alternatives of antibiotic therapy versus watchful waiting and symptomatic relief, is important [57].

The first-line antibiotic of choice for acute bacterial rhinosinusitis is amoxicillin or amoxicillin-clavulanate for 5–10 days. The addition of clavulanate should be considered in patients where bacterial resistance is more likely or in the setting of comorbidities. Examples include recent antibiotic use, failure of prior antibiotic therapy, close contact with children or healthcare environment, smokers, high prevalence of resistant bacteria within the community, elderly, immunocompromised, and diabetics [57, 64, 79, 80]. For penicillin-allergic patients, doxycycline and fluoroquinolones are alternatives [67]. For patients that do not improve after 72 h of antibiotic therapy, the clinician should reassess the patient, and alternative diagnoses should be entertained, including complications of rhinosinusitis. Other disease entities that cause symptoms similar to rhinosinusitis include migraine headache, tension headache, cluster headache, temporal arteritis, dental caries and abscesses, temporomandibular joint dysfunction, allergic rhinitis, preseptal cellulitis, orbital cellulitis, subperiosteal abscess, meningitis, intracranial abscess, osteomyelitis, and cavernous sinus thrombosis. Computed tomography imaging may be helpful if alternative insidious conditions are entertained [57, 64].

Chronic rhinosinusitis is defined as rhinosinusitis that persists unabated for greater than 12 weeks. It is imperative to distinguish recurrent acute rhinosinusitis from chronic rhinosinusitis. The diagnosis of chronic rhinosinusitis should be performed by a specialist using anterior rhinoscopy, nasal endoscopy, or computed tomography and is outside the scope of this chapter. Patients suspected of chronic rhinosinusitis should be referred to an otolaryngologist for further management [57].

References

1. Blaiss MS. Allergic rhinitis: direct and indirect costs. Allergy Asthma Proc. 2010;31:375–80. https://doi.org/10.2500/aap.2010.31.3329.
2. Meltzer EO, Bukstein DA. The economic impact of allergic rhinitis and current guidelines for treatment. Ann Allergy Asthma Immunol. 2011;106:S12–6. https://doi.org/10.1016/j.anai.2010.10.014.
3. Tran NP, Vickery J, Blaiss MS. Management of rhinitis: allergic and non-allergic. Allergy Asthma Immunol Res. 2011;3:148–56. https://doi.org/10.4168/aair.2011.3.3.148.
4. Seidman MD, Gurgel RK, Lin SY, Schwartz SR, Baroody FM, Bonner JR, et al. Clinical practice guideline: allergic rhinitis. Otolaryngol Head Neck Surg. 2015;152:S1–43. https://doi.org/10.1177/0194599814561600.

5. Koinis-Mitchell D, Craig T, Esteban CA, Klein RB. Sleep and allergic disease: a summary of the literature and future directions for research. J Allergy Clin Immunol. 2012;130:1275–81. https://doi.org/10.1016/j.jaci.2012.06.026.
6. Small P, Kim H. Allergic rhinitis. Allergy Asthma Clin Immunol. 2011;7:S3. https://doi.org/10.1186/1710-1492-7-S1-S3.
7. Borish L. Allergic rhinitis: systemic inflammation and implications for management. J Allergy Clin Immunol. 2003;112:1021–31. https://doi.org/10.1016/j.jaci.2003.09.015.
8. Westman M, Stjärne P, Asarnoj A, Kull I, van Hage M, Wickman M, et al. Natural course and comorbidities of allergic and nonallergic rhinitis in children. J Allergy Clin Immunol. 2012;129:403–8. https://doi.org/10.1016/j.jaci.2011.09.036.
9. Kulig M, Klettke U, Wahn V, Forster J, Bauer CP, Wahn U. Development of seasonal allergic rhinitis during the first 7 years of life. J Allergy Clin Immunol. 2000;106:832–9. https://doi.org/10.1067/mai.2000.110098.
10. D'Alonzo GEJ. Scope and impact of allergic rhinitis. J Am Osteopath Assoc. 2002;102:S2–6.
11. Dottorini ML, Bruni B, Peccini F, Bottini P, Pini L, Donato F, et al. Skin prick-test reactivity to aeroallergens and allergic symptoms in an urban population of Central Italy: a longitudinal study. Clin Exp Allergy. 2007;37:188–96. https://doi.org/10.1111/j.1365-2222.2007.02652.x.
12. Kong W, Chen J, Wang Y, Xiang J, Zhang X, Wang J, et al. A population-based 5-year follow-up of allergic rhinitis in Chinese children. Am J Rhinol Allergy. 2012;26:315–20. https://doi.org/10.2500/ajra.2012.26.3790.
13. Kurukulaaratchy RJ, Karmaus W, Arshad SH. Sex and atopy influences on the natural history of rhinitis. Curr Opin Allergy Clin Immunol. 2012;12:7–12. https://doi.org/10.1097/ACI.0b013e32834ecc4e.
14. Yonekura S, Okamoto Y, Horiguchi S, Sakurai D, Chazono H, Hanazawa T, et al. Effects of aging on the natural history of seasonal allergic rhinitis in middle-aged subjects in South Chiba, Japan. Int Arch Allergy Immunol. 2011;157:73–80. https://doi.org/10.1159/000324475.
15. Greiner AN, Hellings PW, Rotiroti G, Scadding GK. Allergic rhinitis. Lancet. 2011;378:2112–22. https://doi.org/10.1016/S0140-6736(11)60130-X.
16. Keil T, Bockelbrink A, Reich A, Hoffmann U, Kamin W, Forster J, et al. The natural history of allergic rhinitis in childhood. Pediatr Allergy Immunol. 2010;21:962–9. https://doi.org/10.1111/j.1399-3038.2010.01046.x.
17. Emanuel MB. Hay fever, a post industrial revolution epidemic: a history of its growth during the 19th century. Clin Exp Allergy. 1988;18:295–304. https://doi.org/10.1111/j.1365-2222.1988.tb02872.x.
18. Okada H, Kuhn C, Feillet H, Bach JF. The "hygiene hypothesis" for autoimmune and allergic diseases: an update. Clin Exp Immunol. 2010;160:1–9. https://doi.org/10.1111/j.1365-2249.2010.04139.x.
19. Yemaneberhan H, Bekele Z, Venn A, Lewis S, Parry E, Britton J. Prevalence of wheeze and asthma and relation to atopy in urban and rural Ethiopia. Lancet. 1997;350:85–90. https://doi.org/10.1016/S0140-6736(97)01151-3.
20. Rees Clayton EM, Todd M, Dowd JB, Aiello AE. The impact of bisphenol A and triclosan on immune parameters in the U.S. population, NHANES 2003–2006. Environ Health Perspect. 2011;119:390–6. https://doi.org/10.1289/ehp.1002883.
21. Baroody F, Naclerio R. Allergic rhinitis. In: Rich R, Fleisher T, Shearer W, et al., editors. Clinical immunology, principles and practice. 2nd ed. London: Mosby; 2001. p. 481.
22. Hansen I, Klimek L, Mösges R, Hörmann K. Mediators of inflammation in the early and the late phase of allergic rhinitis. Curr Opin Allergy Clin Immunol. 2004;4:159–63. https://doi.org/10.1097/00130832-200406000-00004.
23. Orban N, Saleh H, Durham S. Allergic and non-allergic rhinitis. In: Adkinson N, Bochner B, Busse W, et al., editors. Middleton's allergy: principles and practice. 7th ed. St. Louis: Mosby; 2009. p. 973.
24. Eifan AO, Durham SR. Pathogenesis of rhinitis. Clin Exp Allergy. 2016;46:1139–51. https://doi.org/10.1111/cea.12780.

25. Naclerio RM, Proud D, Togias AG, Adkinson NF, Meyers DA, Kagey-Sobotka A, et al. Inflammatory mediators in late antigen-induced rhinitis. N Engl J Med. 1985;313:65–70. https://doi.org/10.1056/nejm198507113130201.
26. McCrory D, Williams J, Dolor R, Gray R, Kolimaga J, Reed S, et al. Management of allergic rhinitis in the working-age population. Evid Rep Technol Assess (Summ). 2003;67:1–4.
27. Bousquet J, Khaltaev N, Cruz AA, Denburg J, Fokkens WJ, Togias A, et al. Allergic Rhinitis and Its Impact on Asthma (ARIA) 2008 update (in collaboration with the World Health Organization, GA2LEN and AllerGen). Allergy. 2008;63:8–160. https://doi.org/10.1111/j.1398-9995.2007.01620.x.
28. Wallace DV, Dykewicz MS, Bernstein DI, Blessing-Moore J, Cox L, Khan DA, et al. The diagnosis and management of rhinitis: an updated practice parameter. J Allergy Clin Immunol. 2008;122:S1–84. https://doi.org/10.1016/j.jaci.2008.06.003.
29. Kiyohara C, Tanaka K, Miyake Y. Genetic susceptibility to atopic dermatitis. Allergol Int. 2008;57:39–56. https://doi.org/10.2332/allergolint.R-07-150.
30. Nayak AS. The asthma and allergic rhinitis link. Allergy Asthma Proc. 2003;24:395–402.
31. Varghese M, Glaum MC, Lockey RF. Drug-induced rhinitis. Clin Exp Allergy. 2010;40:381–4. https://doi.org/10.1111/j.1365-2222.2009.03450.x.
32. Dykewicz MS, Wallace DV, Amrol DJ, Baroody FM, Bernstein JA, Craig TJ, et al. Rhinitis 2020: a practice parameter update. J Allergy Clin Immunol. 2020;146:721–67. https://doi.org/10.1016/j.jaci.2020.07.007.
33. Banov CH, Lieberman P. Efficacy of azelastine nasal spray in the treatment of vasomotor (perennial nonallergic) rhinitis. Ann Allergy Asthma Immunol. 2001;86:28–35. https://doi.org/10.1016/S1081-1206(10)62352-6.
34. Cornelius RS, Martin J, Wippold FJ, Aiken AH, Angtuaco EJ, Berger KL, et al. ACR appropriateness criteria sinonasal disease. J Am Coll Radiol. 2013;10:241–6. https://doi.org/10.1016/j.jacr.2013.01.001.
35. Custovic A, Simpson BM, Simpson A, Kissen P, Woodcock A. Effect of environmental manipulation in pregnancy and early life on respiratory symptoms and atopy during first year of life: a randomised trial. Lancet. 2001;358:188–93. https://doi.org/10.1016/S0140-6736(01)05406-X.
36. Fretzayas A, Kotzia D, Moustaki M. Controversial role of pets in the development of atopy in children. World J Pediatr. 2013;9:112–9. https://doi.org/10.1007/s12519-013-0412-6.
37. Sheikh A, Hurwitz B, Shehata Y. House dust mite avoidance measures for perennial allergic rhinitis. Cochrane Database Syst Rev. 2007;1:CD001563. https://doi.org/10.1002/14651858.CD001563.pub2.
38. Nurmatov U, van Schayck CP, Hurwitz B, Sheikh A. House dust mite avoidance measures for perennial allergic rhinitis: an updated Cochrane systematic review. Allergy. 2012;67:158–65. https://doi.org/10.1111/j.1398-9995.2011.02752.x.
39. Terreehorst I, Oosting AJ, Tempels-Pavlica Z, de Monchy JGR, Bruijnzeel-Koomen CAFM, Hak E, et al. Prevalence and severity of allergic rhinitis in house dust mite-allergic patients with bronchial asthma or atopic dermatitis. Clin Exp Allergy. 2002;32:1160–5. https://doi.org/10.1046/j.1365-2745.2002.01461.x.
40. van Bavel J, Findlay SR, Hampel FC, Martin BG, Ratner P, Field E. Intranasal fluticasone propionate is more effective than terfenadine tablets for seasonal allergic rhinitis. Arch Intern Med. 1994;154:2699–704. https://doi.org/10.1001/archinte.1994.00420230086010.
41. Welsh PW, Stricker WE, Chu CP, Naessens JM, Reese ME, Reed CE, et al. Efficacy of beclomethasone nasal solution, flunisolide, and cromolyn in relieving symptoms of ragweed allergy. Mayo Clin Proc. 1987;62:125–34. https://doi.org/10.1016/S0025-6196(12)61882-5.
42. Kaszuba SM, Baroody FM, deTineo M, Haney L, Blair C, Naclerio RM. Superiority of an intranasal corticosteroid compared with an oral antihistamine in the as-needed treatment of seasonal allergic rhinitis. Arch Intern Med. 2001;161:2581–7. https://doi.org/10.1001/archinte.161.21.2581.
43. Herman H. Once-daily administration of intranasal corticosteroids for allergic rhinitis: a comparative review of efficacy, safety, patient preference, and cost. Am J Rhinol. 2007;21:70–9. https://doi.org/10.2500/ajr.2007.21.2896.

44. Rodrigo GJ, Neffen H. Efficacy of fluticasone furoate nasal spray vs. placebo for the treatment of ocular and nasal symptoms of allergic rhinitis: a systematic review. Clin Exp Allergy. 2011;41:160–70. https://doi.org/10.1111/j.1365-2222.2010.03654.x.
45. Weiner JM, Abramson MJ, Puy RM. Intranasal corticosteroids versus oral H1 receptor antagonists in allergic rhinitis: systematic review of randomised controlled trials. Br Med J. 1998;317:1624–9. https://doi.org/10.1136/bmj.317.7173.1624.
46. Benninger M, Farrar JR, Blaiss M, Chipps B, Ferguson B, Krouse J, et al. Evaluating approved medications to treat allergic rhinitis in the United States: an evidence-based review of efficacy for nasal symptoms by class. Ann Allergy Asthma Immunol. 2010;104:13–29. https://doi.org/10.1016/j.anai.2009.11.020.
47. Brozek JL, Bousquet J, Baena-Cagnani CE, Bonini S, Canonica GW, Casale TB, et al. Allergic rhinitis and its impact on asthma (ARIA) guidelines: 2010 revision. J Allergy Clin Immunol. 2010;126:466–76. https://doi.org/10.1016/j.jaci.2010.06.047.
48. Pullerits T, Praks L, Ristioja V, Lötvall J. Comparison of a nasal glucocorticoid, antileukotriene, and a combination of antileukotriene and antihistamine in the treatment of seasonal allergic rhinitis. J Allergy Clin Immunol. 2002;109:949–55. https://doi.org/10.1067/mai.2002.124467.
49. Horak F, Zieglmayer UP, Zieglmayer R, Kavina A, Marschall K, Munzel U, et al. Azelastine nasal spray and desloratadine tablets in pollen-induced seasonal allergic rhinitis: a pharmacodynamic study of onset of action and efficacy. Curr Med Res Opin. 2006;22:151–7. https://doi.org/10.1185/030079906X80305.
50. Bousquet J, Heinzerling L, Bachert C, Papadopoulos NG, Bousquet PJ, Burney PG, et al. Practical guide to skin prick tests in allergy to aeroallergens. Allergy. 2012;67:18–24. https://doi.org/10.1111/j.1398-9995.2011.02728.x.
51. Bernstein IL, Li JT, Bernstein DI, Hamilton R, Spector SL, Tan R, et al. Allergy diagnostic testing: an updated practice parameter. Ann Allergy Asthma Immunol. 2008;100:S1–148. https://doi.org/10.1016/S1081-1206(10)60305-5.
52. Lucas JW, Schiller JS, Benson V. Summary health statistics for U.S. adults: National Health Interview Survey, 2001. Vital health Stat. 2004;10:1–134.
53. Blackwell DL, Lucas JW, Clarke TC. Summary health statistics for U.S. adults: national health interview survey, 2012. Vital Health Stat. 2014;10:1–161.
54. Bishai WR. Issues in the management of bacterial sinusitis. Otolaryngol Head Neck Surg. 2002;127:S3–9. https://doi.org/10.1067/mhn.2002.130030.
55. Anon JB, et al. Antimicrobial treatment guidelines for acute bacterial rhinosinusitis. Otolaryngol Head Neck Surg. 2004;130:1–45. https://doi.org/10.1016/j.otohns.2003.12.003.
56. Rudmik L, Smith TL, Schlosser RJ, Hwang PH, Mace JC, Soler ZM. Productivity costs in patients with refractory chronic rhinosinusitis. Laryngoscope. 2014;124:2007–12. https://doi.org/10.1002/lary.24630.
57. Rosenfeld RM, Piccirillo JF, Chandrasekhar SS, Brook I, Ashok Kumar K, Kramper M, et al. Clinical practice guideline (update): adult sinusitis executive summary. Otolaryngol Head Neck Surg (United States). 2015;152:598–609. https://doi.org/10.1177/0194599815574247.
58. Hytönen M, Atula T, Pitkäranta A. Complications of acute sinusitis in children. Acta Oto-Laryngol. 2000;120:154–7. https://doi.org/10.1080/000164800454260.
59. Gwaltney JM. Acute community-acquired sinusitis. Clin Infect Dis. 1996;23:1209–23. https://doi.org/10.1093/clinids/23.6.1209.
60. Scheid D, Hamm R. Acute bacterial rhinosinusitis in adults: part I. Evaluation. Am Fam Physician. 2004;70:1685–92.
61. Fokkens WJ, Lund VJ, Mullol J, Bachert C, Alobid I, Baroody F, et al. EPOS 2012: European position paper on rhinosinusitis and nasal polyps 2012. A summary for otorhinolaryngologists. Rhinol J. 2012;50:1–12. https://doi.org/10.4193/Rhino50E2.
62. Piccirillo JF. Acute bacterial sinusitis. N Engl J Med. 2004;351:902–10. https://doi.org/10.1056/NEJMcp035553.
63. Meltzer EO, Hamilos DL. Rhinosinusitis diagnosis and management for the clinician: a synopsis of recent consensus guidelines. Mayo Clin Proc. 2011;86:427–43. https://doi.org/10.4065/mcp.2010.0392.

64. Wald ER, Applegate KE, Bordley C, Darrow DH, Glode MP, Marcy SM, et al. Clinical practice guideline for the diagnosis and management of acute bacterial sinusitis in children aged 1–18 years. Pediatrics. 2013;132:e262–80. https://doi.org/10.1542/peds.2013-1071.
65. Lanza DC, Kennedy DW. Adult rhinosinusitis defined. Otolaryngol Head Neck Surg. 1997;117:S1–7. https://doi.org/10.1016/S0194-5998(97)70001-9.
66. Low DE, Desrosiers M, McSherry J, Garber G, Williams JW Jr, Remy H, et al. A practical guide for the diagnosis and treatment of acute sinusitis. CMAJ. 1997;156(Suppl 6):S1–14.
67. Chow AW, Benninger MS, Brook I, Brozek JL, Goldstein EJC, Hicks LA, et al. Executive summary: IDSA clinical practice guideline for acute bacterial rhinosinusitis in children and adults. Clin Infect Dis. 2012;54:1041–5. https://doi.org/10.1093/cid/cir1043.
68. Lacroix JS, Ricchetti A, Lew D, Delhumeau C, Morabia A, Stalder H, et al. Symptoms and clinical and radiological signs predicting the presence of pathogenic bacteria in acute rhinosinusitis. Acta Otolaryngol. 2002;122:192–6. https://doi.org/10.1080/00016480252814216.
69. Williams JW, Simel DL, Roberts L, Samsa GP. Clinical evaluation for sinusitis: making the diagnosis by history and physical examination. Ann Intern Med. 1992;117:705–10. https://doi.org/10.7326/0003-4819-117-9-705.
70. Hauer AJ, Luiten EL, van Erp NF, Blase PE, Aarts MCJ, Kaper NM, et al. No evidence for distinguishing bacterial from viral acute rhinosinusitis using fever and facial/dental pain: a systematic review of the evidence base. Otolaryngol Head Neck Surg (United States). 2014;150:28–33. https://doi.org/10.1177/0194599813510891.
71. Setzen G, Ferguson BJ, Han JK, Rhee JS, Cornelius RS, Froum SJ, et al. Clinical consensus statement: appropriate use of computed tomography for paranasal sinus disease. Otolaryngol Head Neck Surg (United States). 2012;147:808–16. https://doi.org/10.1177/0194599812463848.
72. deShazo RD, Chapin K, Swain RE. Fungal sinusitis. N Engl J Med. 1997;337:254–9. https://doi.org/10.1056/NEJM199707243370407.
73. Mylonakis E, Rich J, Skolnik PR, de Orchis DF, Flanigan T. Invasive aspergillus sinusitis in patients with human immunodeficiency virus infection report of 2 cases and review. Medicine. 1997;76:249–55. https://doi.org/10.1097/00005792-199707000-00003.
74. Monroe MM, McLean M, Sautter N, Wax MK, Andersen PE, Smith TL, et al. Invasive fungal rhinosinusitis: a 15-year experience with 29 patients. Laryngoscope. 2013;123:1583–7. https://doi.org/10.1002/lary.23978.
75. Aribandi M, McCoy VA, Bazan C. Imaging features of invasive and noninvasive fungal sinusitis: a review. Radiographics. 2007;27:1283–96. https://doi.org/10.1148/rg.275065189.
76. DelGaudio JM, Swain RE, Kingdom TT, Muller S, Hudgins PA. Computed tomographic findings in patients with invasive fungal sinusitis. Arch Otolaryngol Head Neck Surg. 2003;129:236–40. https://doi.org/10.1001/archotol.129.2.236.
77. Arroll B, Kenealy T. Antibiotics for the common cold and acute purulent rhinitis. Cochrane Database Syst Rev. 2005;3:CD000247. https://doi.org/10.1002/14651858.cd000247.pub2.
78. Arroll B, Kenealy T. Are antibiotics effective for acute purulent rhinitis? Systematic review and meta-analysis of placebo controlled randomised trials. BMJ. 2006;333:279. https://doi.org/10.1136/bmj.38891.681215.AE.
79. Jenkins SG, Farrell DJ, Patel M, Lavin BS. Trends in anti-bacterial resistance among *Streptococcus pneumoniae* isolated in the USA, 2000–2003: PROTEKT US years 1–3. J Infect. 2005;51:355–63. https://doi.org/10.1016/j.jinf.2005.04.015.
80. Brook I, Gober AE. Resistance to antimicrobials used for therapy of otitis media and sinusitis: effect of previous antimicrobial therapy and smoking. Ann Otol Rhinol Laryngol. 1999;108:645–7. https://doi.org/10.1177/000348949910800704.

Neck Pain

7

Michael Seth Smith

7.1 Introduction

Neck pain is a common complaint among patients, with up to two-thirds of people experiencing this malady at some point in their lives [1]. In the United States in 2010, neck pain led to 16.3 million patient visits, 5% of which were emergency department visits [2]. The majority of patients presenting with neck pain do not require hospitalization, indicating that most people presenting with neck pain may be safely managed in the outpatient setting. It is well known that many patients, especially those of lower socioeconomic status, will seek nonemergency care in the emergency department [3]. Although these patients will not likely require admission when they present with neck pain, the differential diagnosis of neck pain does contain serious and even life-threatening etiologies of which the emergency physician must be cognizant.

Neck pain can be a manifestation of a wide variety of medical conditions besides musculoskeletal or soft tissue injuries [4]. Careful history taking and physical examination, when coupled with a high index of suspicion in the appropriate cases, will allow the emergency physician to triage patients with neck pain into low- and high-risk categories. Low-risk patients can be managed in the outpatient setting, while high-risk patients may warrant admission and additional specialized consultations.

7.2 Risk Factors for Neck Pain

- Participation in contact sports or other activities predisposing to acute injury [5].
- Presence of underlying medical conditions which can manifest as neck pain.

M. S. Smith (✉)
Division of Sports Medicine, Department of Orthopedics and Rehabilitation, University of Florida, Gainesville, FL, USA

B. K. Desai et al. (eds.), *Primary Care for Emergency Physicians*,
https://doi.org/10.1007/978-3-031-64676-8_7

- Poor posture, postural awareness, and/or ergonomics.
- Psychosocial factors, including occupational history and presence of underlying psychologic disorders or poor coping skills.
- Advancing age.

7.3 Differential Diagnosis

The differential diagnosis of neck pain is broad, involving the musculoskeletal structures of the neck as well as other organs which can refer pain to the neck. The following list is not comprehensive but rather representative of the multiple etiologies of neck pain.

- Traumatic.
  - Cervical paraspinal muscular strain or cervical ligamentous sprain.
    For example, classic "whiplash" injury from forced cervical flexion and extension resulting in tension-compression forces in the cervical spine [6].
    Can be immediate onset or delayed in presentation from when injury actually occurred.
  - Noncontact fractures.
    For example, clay-shoveler's fracture [5, 7]
  - Fractures secondary to impact or contact [5, 8]
- Nontraumatic
  - Musculoskeletal
    Cervical spine osteoarthritis
    - Poor correlation between radiographic findings and patient complaints [9].

    Longus colli tendinitis/retropharyngeal calcific tendinitis.
    - Most common symptoms are acute onset of neck pain, odynophagia, and/or reduced ROM.
    - Benign but difficult to distinguish from retropharyngeal abscess [10, 11].

    Diffuse idiopathic skeletal hyperostosis (DISH).
    - Cervical spine involvement found in up to 76% of patients with DISH.
    - Can be complicated by dysphagia, hoarseness, and stridor depending on which local structures are affected [12, 13].

    Cervical intervertebral disk herniation.
    Thoracic outlet syndrome.
    Myofascial trigger points.
    Wry neck.
    - Zygapophyseal: associated with sudden movements and acute pain, more common in younger population.
    - Diskogenic: associated with more chronic course, more common in older population [14].

    Referred shoulder pain.

- Rotator cuff tendinitis/impingement syndrome.
- Adhesive capsulitis.

– Infectious.

Infectious thyroiditis.

Pharyngitis.

- Need to distinguish bacterial from viral infections and treat bacterial infections to prevent complications [15]

Deep space infections (retropharyngeal or precervical infections).

- Must look for an underlying cause as most retropharyngeal abscesses occur in the setting of immunodeficiency or injury by a foreign body [16].

Diskitis/osteomyelitis.

- More common in patients older than 50 years.
- Risk factors include intravenous drug abuse, chronic hemodialysis, and other immunocompromising states [17]

Lymphadenitis.

- Should prompt evaluation into infectious etiologies affecting the head and neck [18]

Herpes zoster.

- Pain can present several days prior to onset of rash leading to incorrect or delayed diagnosis [19].

– Cardiovascular.

Carotid artery dissection.

- May not always be associated with typical cardiovascular risk factors but can be a sequela of neck injury, including chiropractic manipulation [20]
- Can be associated with focal neurologic signs, including amaurosis fugax, partial Horner's syndrome, and visual field disturbances [21]

Spontaneous hematoma.

- Possibly arising secondary to use of multiple blood-thinning agents prescribed for cardiovascular indications [22]

Myocardial infarction (referred pain).

- In one study, approximately 25% of patients with an acute myocardial infarction experienced neck pain, with no significant difference between male and female patients [23].

– Rheumatologic.

Rheumatoid arthritis (RA).

- Neck pain is prevalent in 43–86% of patients with RA, with radiographic changes noted in greater than 80% of patients [24].

Ankylosing spondylitis (AS).

- Neck pain was found to be a presenting symptom of AS in approximately 27% of men and 33% of women [25].

Autoimmune thyroiditis.

– Metabolic.

Gout/pseudogout.

- Cervical spine tophi formation, though unusual, can be seen in advanced cases of untreated hyperuricemia and gout.
- An MRI may be helpful in establishing the diagnosis as the clinical picture can mimic rheumatoid arthritis [26].

  Paget's disease.
- Neurologic.

  Chiari I malformation.
  - Neck pain is a common presenting symptom in patients with Chiari I malformation with neck trauma being a common trigger in children with acute presentation [27, 28].

  Cervicogenic headache.
- Visceral.

  Esophageal dysmotility/obstruction.

  Referred visceral pain.
  - Autonomic dysfunction, changes in diaphragmatic pressure, and/or peritoneal irritation, as is seen in disorders of varying viscera, can lead to "phrenic pain" or referred pain along C3/C4 dermatomes [29].

7.4 Red Flags of Neck Pain

Red flags of neck pain include the five D's [14]:

1. Dizziness
2. Diplopia
3. Dysphagia
4. Dysarthria
5. Drop attacks

The presence of these symptoms should alert the emergency physician to the possibility of cardiovascular etiologies such as vertebrobasilar insufficiency or carotid artery dissection.

7.5 History

The wide differential diagnosis of neck pain can be narrowed based on the history obtained from the patient. Obtaining a detailed and comprehensive history will not only help with diagnosis but also with treatment plans. Pertinent information to gather while taking a history includes but is not limited to:

- Symptom onset
  - Acute versus insidious/chronic
- Location of pain
  - Localized versus diffuse

- Presence of additional symptoms
  - Headache
  - Radiating neuropathic pain
  - Red flags (five D's as listed above)
- Aggravating and alleviating factors, including medications and other treatment modalities
- Occupational or recreational factors

7.6 Physical Examination

As with physical examination of any other area of the body, history obtained from the patient or witness will guide the physical examination. An abrupt onset of symptoms following a traumatic event would lead the examiner to look for acute musculoskeletal injuries, whereas an insidious onset of symptoms would prompt the examiner to look for alternative explanations for the patient's complaints. If the cause of pain is thought to be structural, initial evaluation should focus on determining whether the pain generator in question is articular, muscular, or neural in nature [14].

- Vital signs
  - The presence of fever should prompt a search for an infectious etiology of symptoms
- Inspection of skin and examination of musculoskeletal structures
  - Presence of skin abnormalities such as rashes, erythema/discoloration, swelling, etc., could alter differential diagnosis
  - Examination of contour (back to wall test):
    Loss of normal cervical lordosis can be caused by ankylosing spondylitis, degenerative changes of the cervical spine, injury to the soft tissue, etc.
  - Palpation of vertebral bodies, paraspinal musculature, upper trapezius, and sternocleidomastoids.
  - Assess range of motion in six directions:
    Flexion/extension
    Rotation
    Side bending
  - Special testing:
    Spurling maneuver (neck compression test).
    - Used to identify lateral rupture of a cervical intravertebral disk causing nerve root compression.

    Roos test and Adson's test.
    - Used to evaluate for thoracic outlet syndrome in patients presenting with neck pain in conjunction with numbness and tingling of an upper limb.
  - Neurologic exam if patient presents with radiation of symptoms below the shoulder.

- Examination of other structures in the neck as indicated by history.
  - Visual examination of oropharyngeal structures.
  - Palpate thyroid:
    May be able to auscultate a bruit in hyperthyroidism.
  - Palpate posterior and anterior cervical lymph nodes:
    Preauricular, postauricular, and occipital nodes are usually visible if significantly involved in underlying process [30].

7.7 Introduction to Treatment

Much as the physical examination will be guided by the history of present injury, so will treatment options be directed by the nature of the underlying process. Neck pain caused by non-musculoskeletal pathology should be treated as indicated to address the underlying process (i.e., treating an infection, myocardial infarction, etc.). The following are some broad principles for treatment of both acute and chronic musculoskeletal neck pain:

- Acute/traumatic musculoskeletal injury
  - In trauma patients, one must decide which patients require imaging of the cervical spine. The NEXUS low-risk criteria are a validated model that can assist the emergency physician in decision-making [31].

NEXUS low-risk criteria
No tenderness at posterior midline of C-spine
No focal neurologic deficit
Normal level of alertness
No evidence of intoxication
No distracting injury

  - Fractures involving multiple levels, involving C3–C5, or demonstrating widened disk space or facet dislocation on plain films should be evaluated for adjacent level ligamentous injury (ALLI) by MRI [32].
  - Less serious acute musculoskeletal injuries (e.g., whiplash) can often be managed symptomatically with short courses of acetaminophen, nonsteroidal anti-inflammatories, and muscle relaxants.
- Musculoskeletal injury of a chronic nature
  - Acute injury, such as whiplash, can turn into a chronic pain syndrome.
  - Most chronic neck pain treatment plans will require a multimodality/multidisciplinary approach including:
    Patient education, including expected outcomes.
    Physical therapy with postural rehabilitation, muscle strength, and control techniques.
    Medications for short durations.
    Referral to psychology/psychiatry as needed.

Invasive procedures (corticosteroid injections, surgical intervention) but only when an adequate amount of conservative management has failed.

7.8 Pharmacologic Treatment

The pharmacologic treatment options listed below assume that the patient's condition does not warrant admission to the hospital and can be managed conservatively.

- Acute musculoskeletal injury.
  - Acetaminophen.

    Acts as an analgesic and antipyretic on cannabinoid receptors in the central nervous system.

    Dosed 650–1000 mg every 8 h as needed, maximum daily dose 3000 mg (FDA reduced this recommended maximum dose from 4000 mg in 2014). No benefit seen from taking doses higher than 1000 mg at a time [14].

    Pitfalls.

    1. Prescribing acetaminophen when a patient is already taking acetaminophen-containing medications such as oxycodone-acetaminophen. Patients must be counseled that 3000 mg of acetaminophen from all sources counts toward the maximum daily limit.
    2. Prescribing to patients with liver injury.
    3. Unlikely to alleviate severe pain.
  - Nonsteroidal anti-inflammatory drugs (NSAIDs)

Commonly prescribed NSAIDs	Typical dosing
Ibuprofen	400–800 mg PO every 4–6 h
Meloxicam	7.5–15 mg PO every 24 h
Diclofenac	25–50 mg PO every 8–12 h
Naproxen	250–1000 mg PO every 12–24 h

Inhibit cyclooxygenase (COX) enzyme which has a role in the inflammatory cascade after acute injury. Antithrombotic effects are seen in addition to analgesic and antipyretic effects.

There is evidence that NSAIDs are more efficacious than placebo for the treatment of neck pain [33].

Pitfalls:

1. Prescribing a prolonged course (>5 days) [14].
2. Prescribing to patients at risk for peptic ulcer disease without co-prescribing a PPI or H2 blocker.
3. Prescribing to patients with history of renal insufficiency.
4. Prescribing to patients with elevated risk of cardiovascular disease.
5. Prescribing to patients with NSAID allergy.
6. Skeletal muscle relaxants.

Commonly prescribed muscle relaxants	Typical dosing
Cyclobenzaprine	5–10 mg PO every 8 h as needed
Methocarbamol	1500 mg PO every 6 h for 2–3 days with maximum dose 8000 mg/day and then reduce to 4000 mg/day
Carisoprodol	250–350 mg PO every 8 h and at hour of sleep

Related to cyclic antidepressants, have multiple effects on neurotransmitter pathways resulting in sedation.

One study showed that there was no benefit in pain control in prescribing NSAIDs plus muscle relaxants versus NSAIDs alone, but there was a higher rate of nervous system complications because of the central action of muscle relaxants [34].

Pitfalls:

1. Skeletal muscle relaxants cause sedation as a class effect; patients must be cautioned about sedation as a probable side effect.
2. Cyclobenzaprine should not be prescribed to patients:
   - Who are taking or have taken a MAO inhibitor within the past 14 days.
   - Who have hyperthyroidism.
   - Who are recovering from a myocardial infarction, have cardiac conduction abnormalities, or have congestive heart failure.
3. The dose of methocarbamol should be reduced in patients with hepatic impairment.

- Chronic musculoskeletal pain.
  – Acetaminophen, NSAIDs, and muscle relaxants should be prescribed at the lowest possible effective dose and for the shortest duration possible. They should not play a role in chronic musculoskeletal neck pain due to the adverse effects of long-term administration.

References

1. Binder AI. Cervical spondylosis and neck pain. Bmj. 2007;334(7592):527–31.
2. United States Bone and Joint Initiative. Summary of resource allocation of total health care occurrences for back pain and related conditions by sex, United States 2010. http://www.boneandjointburden.org/docs/T2.4.1.pdf. Accessed 17 Nov 2015.
3. Wexler R, Hefner JL, Sieck C, et al. Connecting emergency department patients to primary care. J Am Board Fam Med. 2015;28(6):722–32.
4. Kazeminasab S, Nejadghaderi SA, Amiri P, et al. Neck pain: global epidemiology, trends and risk factors. BMC Musculoskelet Disord. 2022;23(1):26.
5. Paulus S, Kennedy DJ. Return to play considerations for cervical spine injuries in athletes. Phys Med Rehabil Clin N Am. 2014;25(4):723–33.
6. Erbulut DU. Biomechanics of neck injuries resulting from rear-end vehicle collisions. Turk Neurosurg. 2014;24(4):466–70.
7. Akhaddar A, El-asri A, Boucetta M. Multiple isolated thoracic spinous process fractures (Clay-Shoveler's fracture). Spine J. 2011;11(5):458–9.

8. Marcon RM, Cristante AF, Teixeira WJ, Narasaki DK, Oliveira RP, de Barros Filho TE. Fractures of the cervical spine. Clinics (Sao Paulo). 2013;68(11):1455–61.
9. Rudy IS, Poulos A, Owen L, et al. The correlation of radiographic findings and patient symptomatology in cervical degenerative joint disease: a cross-sectional study. Chiropr Man Ther. 2015;23:9.
10. Gabra N, Belair M, Ayad T. Retropharyngeal calcific tendinitis mimicking a retropharyngeal phlegmon. Case Rep Otolaryngol. 2013;2013:912628.
11. Mannoji C, Koda M, Furuya T, Aramomi M. Calcific tendinitis of the longus Colli. Intern Med. 2015;54(12):1573.
12. Hermann KG, Bollow M. Rethinking diffuse idiopathic skeletal hyperostosis. Rheumatology (Oxford). 2014;53:1917–9.
13. Mader R. Clinical manifestations of diffuse idiopathic skeletal hyperostosis of the cervical spine. Semin Arthritis Rheum. 2002;32(2):130–5.
14. Brukner P, Khan K. Brukner and Khan's clinical sports medicine. 4th ed. New York: McGraw-Hill; 2012.
15. Noh HJ, de Freitas CA, de Paula ESFSR, Simoes JC, Kosugi EM. Lemierre syndrome: a rare complication of pharyngotonsillitis. Braz J Otorhinolaryngol. 2015;81(5):568–70.
16. Schott CK, Counselman FL, Ashe AR. A pain in the neck: non-traumatic adult retropharyngeal abscess. J Emerg Med. 2013;44(2):329–31.
17. Berbari EF, Kanj SS, Kowalski TJ, et al. Executive summary: 2015 Infectious Diseases Society of America (IDSA) clinical practice guidelines for the diagnosis and treatment of native vertebral osteomyelitis in adults. Clin Infect Dis. 2015;61(6):859–63.
18. Gosche JR, Vick L. Acute, subacute, and chronic cervical lymphadenitis in children. Semin Pediatr Surg. 2006;15(2):99–106.
19. Johnson RW, Alvarez-Pasquin MJ, Bijl M, Franco E, Gaillat J, Clara JG, Labetoulle M, Michel JP, Naldi L, Sanmarti LS, Weinke T. Herpes zoster epidemiology, management, and disease and economic burden in Europe: a multidisciplinary perspective [Erratum in: Ther Adv Vaccines. 2016 Jan;4(1–2):32.]. Ther Adv Vaccines. 2015;3(4):109–20.
20. Thomas LC. Cervical arterial dissection: an overview and implications for manipulative therapy practice. Man Ther. 2016;21:2–9.
21. Guillon B, Lévy C, Bousser MG. Internal carotid artery dissection: an update. J Neurol Sci. 1998;153(2):146–58.
22. Shirakura Y, Fukuoka T. Man with sudden neck pain. J Emerg Med. 2015;49(6):e199–200.
23. Berg J, Bjorck L, Dudas K, Lappas G, Rosengren A. Symptoms of a first acute myocardial infarction in women and men. Gend Med. 2009;6(3):454–62.
24. Gillick JL, Wainwright J, Das K. Rheumatoid arthritis and the cervical spine a review on the role of surgery. Int J Rheumatol. 2015;2015:252456.
25. Roussou E, Sultana S. Spondyloarthritis in women: differences in disease onset, clinical presentation, and Bath Ankylosing Spondylitis Disease Activity and Functional indices (BASDAI and BASFI) between men and women with spondyloarthritides. Clin Rheumatol. 2011;30(1):121–7.
26. Nunes EA, Rosseti AG Jr, Ribeiro DS, Santiago M. Gout initially mimicking rheumatoid arthritis and later cervical spine involvement. Case Rep Rheumatol. 2014;2014:357826.
27. Aitken LA, Lindan CE, Sidney S, et al. Chiari type I malformation in a pediatric population. Pediatr Neurol. 2009;40(6):449–54.
28. Talamonti G, Marcati E, Gribaudi G, Picano M, D'Aliberti G. Acute presentation of Chiari 1 malformation in children. Childs Nerv Syst. 2020;36(5):899–909.
29. Oliva-Pascual-Vaca Á, González-González C, Oliva-Pascual-Vaca J, et al. Visceral origin: an underestimated source of neck pain. A systematic scoping review. Diagnostics (Basel). 2019;9(4):186.
30. Orient JM, Sapira JD. Sapira's art and science of bedside diagnosis. 3rd ed. Philadelphia: Lippincott Williams & Wilkins; 2005.

31. Hoffman JR, Mower WR, Wolfson AB, Todd KH, Zucker MI. Validity of a set of clinical criteria to rule out injury to the cervical spine in patients with blunt trauma. National Emergency X-Radiography Utilization Study Group. N Engl J Med. 2000;343(2):94–9.
32. Awad BI, Carmody MA, Lubelski D, et al. Adjacent level ligamentous injury associated with traumatic cervical spine fractures: indications for imaging and implications for treatment. World Neurosurg. 2015;84(1):69–75.
33. Wong JJ, Côté P, Ameis A, et al. Are non-steroidal anti-inflammatory drugs effective for the management of neck pain and associated disorders, whiplash-associated disorders, or non-specific low back pain? A systematic review of systematic reviews by the Ontario Protocol for Traffic Injury Management (OPTIMa) Collaboration. Eur Spine J. 2016;25(1):34–61.
34. Turturro MA, Frater CR, D'Amico FJ. Cyclobenzaprine with ibuprofen versus ibuprofen alone in acute myofascial strain: a randomized, double-blind clinical trial. Ann Emerg Med. 2003;41(6):818–26.

Dysphagia and Odynophagia

8

Elisabeth H. W. Hwang and Charles Hwang

8.1 Dysphagia

Dysphagia is a common problem encountered by primary care physicians and will impact the care of patients in any healthcare setting. Dysphagia occurs in up to 30–40% of patients in long-term care facilities and up to 50% of elderly patients or patients with neurological conditions; it approaches 80% in patients with neurological diseases such as TBI and Parkinson's disease [1–3]. It is a potentially life-threatening process that may cause food impaction, airway obstruction, aspiration pneumonia, dehydration, weight loss, and nutritional deficiencies [4, 5].

Swallowing is divided into two main phases, an oropharyngeal phase and an esophageal phase. The location of dysphagia is important because the potential pathology, and subsequent evaluation and management, varies by anatomical location.

Swallowing is mediated by a complex mechanism involving the cerebrum, brainstem, and cranial nerves. It requires coordination between striated and smooth muscle, which are innervated by the somatic and autonomic (enteric) nervous systems, respectively [6]. During the *oral* phase, the muscles of the mouth and tongue masticate and prepare a food bolus by pushing the food against the palate. This phase of eating is under conscious control. Once food enters the palatoglossal arch, the first irreversible step of swallowing, the *pharyngeal* phase, occurs. The pharyngeal phase is involuntary and involves the larynx, pharynx, and esophagus creating coordinated contractions to propel the food bolus through the upper esophageal sphincter (UES). Ordinarily, the airway is protected during this phase by the closure of the vocal cords and movement of the epiglottis to cover the larynx. The *esophageal* phase consists of autonomous peristalsis of the food bolus through the esophagus and,

E. H. W. Hwang · C. Hwang (✉)
Department of Emergency Medicine, University of Florida College of Medicine, Gainesville, FL, USA
e-mail: hwang.c@ufl.edu

B. K. Desai et al. (eds.), *Primary Care for Emergency Physicians*,
https://doi.org/10.1007/978-3-031-64676-8_8

ultimately, relaxation of the lower esophageal sphincter (LES) to allow for passage of the bolus into the stomach [7].

8.1.1 Pathophysiology

Dysphagia is objectively defined as the abnormal transit of solids and/or liquids from the mouth to the hypopharynx or through the esophagus [8, 9]. Subjectively, patients experience the sensation of a delay in transit. The subjective sensation and objective findings of dysphagia may be congruent or disproportionate; for example, patients with functional dysphagia may experience the sensation of transit delay despite objectively normal transit. Conversely, patients with decreased esophageal sensation may have true dysphagia but may not perceive the severity of their symptoms [8].

Dysphagia can be categorized based on the phase of swallowing that is perturbed. *Oropharyngeal dysphagia* typically involves broad multisystem musculoskeletal and nervous system pathology and affects three main populations—elderly patients, patients with neurological diseases, and patients with head and neck diseases. Examples of neurologic pathologies include stroke, dementia, Parkinson's disease, myasthenia gravis, multiple sclerosis, botulism, progressive supranuclear palsy, polymyositis, amyotrophic lateral sclerosis, muscular dystrophy, and cerebral palsy, among other neuromuscular diseases. Local anatomic pathologies include abscess, neoplasm, thyromegaly, cervical hyperostosis, Zenker's diverticulum, postsurgical or radiation-related changes, and ingestion of caustic substances [2–4, 8–10].

Esophageal dysphagia refers to abnormal transit during the esophageal phase of swallowing, which can be further categorized into structural and motor abnormalities. Structural abnormalities primarily result from pathologies that narrow the esophageal lumen (e.g., Schatzki's rings, esophagitis, head and neck or esophageal neoplasms, peptic strictures, or extrinsic compression of the esophagus by lymphadenopathy or cancer). The luminal diameter of a normal adult esophagus is 2–3 cm; luminal diameters less than 1.3 cm can manifest in solid food esophageal dysphagia because this diameter is smaller than the typical food boluses created by the action of the mouth and tongue. Motor pathologies can affect the peristaltic wave that propels food down the esophagus or cause inappropriate sphincter relaxation preventing entry of food into the stomach [2, 4, 8–10]. Refer to Table 8.1 for causes of esophageal dysphagia.

The two most common causes of obstructive structural lesions are *Schatzki's rings* (located at the squamocolumnar junction) and *esophageal webs* (located in the upper esophagus). Both are thin membranous structures that obstruct the esophageal lumen. Boluses of solid food cannot smoothly pass these obstructing membranes, causing food impaction and resulting in dysphagia with associated symptoms of heartburn and chest pain [2]. *Esophageal strictures* and *esophagitis* develop from esophageal inflammation that ultimately results in fibrosis. Inflammatory causes of esophagitis may include peptic diseases, autoimmune diseases, infection, ingestion of caustic medications or substances, trauma, and radiation [2]. Infectious causes of

Table 8.1 Esophageal dysphagia

Structural causes	Motor causes
• Peptic stricture • Zenker's diverticulum • Schatzki's ring • Esophageal web • Esophagitis • Aortic compression • Lymphadenopathy • Radiation-induced stricture • Esophageal adenocarcinoma • Squamous cell carcinoma • Caustic medications or ingestions (e.g., bisphosphonates, tetracycline, NSAIDs)	• Achalasia • Nutcracker esophagus • Diffuse esophageal spasm • Scleroderma • Functional

esophagitis are typically those associated with immunosuppression, such as human immunodeficiency virus (HIV)/acquired immunodeficiency syndrome (AIDS), *Candida albicans*, herpes simplex virus (HSV), cytomegalovirus (CMV), varicella zoster virus (VZV), and Epstein-Barr virus (EBV). *Zenker's diverticulum* is a herniation of the pharyngeal mucosa through the Killian triangle, a triangular-shaped region of weakness in the pharyngeal muscular wall, which can cause regurgitation of food, halitosis, and dysphagia of solid and liquid foods. Finally, *esophageal malignancies* are characterized by the progressive dysphagia of solids to liquids over several weeks to months, accompanied by weight loss, anorexia, and anemia. Risk factors include smoking, alcohol abuse, and long-standing history of reflux [2].

Any disease that causes abnormal peristalsis will cause dysphagia secondary to motor dysfunction. *Achalasia* is caused by the loss of inhibitory myenteric plexus neurons that facilitate LES relaxation. This causes abnormal contraction and relaxation of esophageal smooth muscle, resulting in elevated LES pressure and absence of distal esophageal peristalsis. Achalasia results in the stasis and regurgitation of ingested foods, the dilatation of the distal esophagus, and progressive liquid and solid food dysphagia that can result in coughing, aspiration, weight loss, and heartburn [2, 11]. *Nutcracker esophagus* is the most common esophageal motility disorder, accounting for more than 40% of esophageal motility disorders. In this disorder, peristalsis is coordinated but of excessive amplitude, resulting in chest pain [2]. *Diffuse esophageal spasm* is characterized by uncoordinated contractions rather than smooth peristalsis, preventing the normal forward transit of food. Symptoms are usually intermittent and can include globus sensation, heartburn, and regurgitation [2].

8.1.2 History

A careful history is of paramount importance in identifying the type, location, and etiology of dysphagia and helps to guide evaluation and treatment [4, 10]. Important historical elements to elucidate include onset, type of food, duration, severity, localization, progression, associated symptoms, and alleviating and exacerbating factors including food consistencies and present diet. A broad differential is imperative as dysphagia is not limited to the gastrointestinal tract; for example, motor pathology may be caused by cranial nerve defects (pertinent questions include drooling, voice change, aspiration), and structural pathologies are varied (Table 8.1) [2, 4, 8].

Patients with oropharyngeal dysphagia have difficulty *initiating* swallowing, with associated symptoms of coughing, choking, drooling, regurgitation, and aspiration. Symptoms are localized to the oropharynx or hypopharynx. History of head and neck surgery or radiation, previous diagnosis of head and neck cancer, stroke, and neurological disorders are important elements of the past medical history. As a result of their symptoms, patients may change their dietary habits, resulting in unexpected weight loss [4, 5, 8].

Patients with esophageal dysphagia experience food "sticking" in the throat, upper chest, suprasternal notch, or retrosternal area *after* swallowing. Constant dysphagia with solids and liquids is suggestive of motor pathology as the neuromuscular peristalsis affects both solids and liquids. Conversely, intermittent dysphagia with solids is suggestive of structural abnormalities. The principal symptoms of structural/anatomic causes of dysphagia occur primarily with ingestion of solids and not liquids; symptoms are aggravated with larger and denser solids [4, 8]. Progressive dysphagia over an extended period of weeks to months raises concern for neoplasms, whereas dysphagia that is episodic and unchanged over years suggests a benign disease process such as Schatzki's rings or esophagitis. Of note, the location and severity of solid food dysphagia is not necessarily proportional to the severity of luminal narrowing, as patients can modify and adapt their dietary habits to accommodate their dysphagia by avoiding certain foods, chewing foods fully, and mixing liquids with their solid meals [4, 8].

Chest pain or discomfort and heartburn frequently accompany dysphagia regardless of its etiology. Cardiac causes of chest pain (acute coronary syndrome) should be ruled out before evaluating the patient for causes of dysphagia [2]. Associated odynophagia suggests inflammation in the upper gastrointestinal tract; common causes include infection, medication-induced, or ulceration. Any immune system suppression can cause infectious esophagitis, and patients may have concurrent cardiac, respiratory, or abdominal symptoms of immunosuppression [2].

Various foods, toxins, and medications can cause direct mucosal injury or decrease LES tone. A patient with new onset of symptoms should be evaluated to determine if a medication is the culprit; side effects of these medications may contribute to their symptoms of dysphagia. Table 8.2 contains a list of medications, foods, and toxins that can cause or worsen dysphagia [2–5].

Past medical history may include autoimmune diseases, such as CREST syndrome which is associated with scleroderma. Patients with a history of gastritis, reflux, peptic ulcer disease, or caustic ingestion can have esophagitis or peptic strictures [2].

Other important considerations in eliciting a history include asking about compensatory and adaptation mechanisms that patients may develop to mitigate their

Table 8.2 Medications and toxins that can affect swallowing

Sedation • Benzodiazepines • Barbiturates • Neuroleptics • Anticonvulsants Myopathy • HMG-CoA reductase inhibitors (statins) • Corticosteroids Impaired motility • Anticholinergics • Calcium channel blockers • Beta-blockers • Nitrates • Botulinum toxin • Phenothiazines • Amiodarone • Procainamide Foods • Alcohol • Chocolate • Peppermint • Onion	Xerostomia • Anticholinergics • Antihypertensives • Antihistamines • Antipsychotics • Anxiolytics • Antidepressants • Anticonvulsants • Antiparkinsonian agents • Narcotics Inflammation • Antibacterial agents such as tetracycline, doxycycline, clindamycin, trimethoprim-sulfamethoxazole, erythromycin • Iron • Nonsteroidal anti-inflammatory drugs and aspirin • Corticosteroids • Bisphosphonates • Zidovudine • Quinidine • Chemotherapeutic agents

symptoms. For example, patients may avoid certain foods, eat slower, and be the last to finish a meal to decrease the severity of their dysphagia or learn to drink fluids with solids to facilitate transit [2, 8, 9]. Ultimately, patients with food aversion or decreased oral intake may experience unexpected weight loss and dehydration [8].

8.1.3 Physical Exam

The examination may elucidate the cause of dysphagia. The primary goals of the physical examination are to (1) identify underlying systemic or metabolic disorders, (2) identify neurological disorders and their severity, and (3) identify sequelae of dysphagia, including dehydration, metabolic derangements, or respiratory/pulmonary compromise. Therefore, the physical exam should include the head and neck, mouth, oropharynx, larynx, cardiopulmonary and nervous systems, and cranial nerves [5, 8].

Initial vital signs may demonstrate fever, tachycardia, tachypnea, or hypoxia if there is infection, airway obstruction, dehydration, or respiratory distress secondary to dysphagia or one of its complications. The neurological exam should be centered around the suspected pathology, namely, to assess the mental status for signs of cognitive dysfunction and to identify cranial nerve deficits, proximal or asymmetric extremity weakness, fasciculations, reflexes, dysarthria, dysphonia, glossal atrophy, and tremors [2, 8]. The neurological assessment may identify impaired cognition, focal neurologic deficits consistent with stroke, or other chronic illnesses that affect neurologic function.

The head and neck examination is necessary to evaluate dentition, oropharyngeal lesions, glossal fasciculations, signs of dehydration, palatal or uvular or glossal deviation, thyromegaly, and lymphadenopathy [2, 8]. Evaluate the abdomen for tenderness and masses. Positive fecal occult blood testing may indicate neoplastic disease or severe esophagitis. The skin may demonstrate changes of autoimmune or connective tissue diseases, such as scleroderma which would manifest with skin thickening and decreased joint mobility in the hands [2].

One of the easiest and most important parts of the physical exam is to watch the patient swallow. Oftentimes, patients may not recognize the causes or severity of their difficulty in swallowing. Observation of swallowing may provide information with respect to the degree of dysphagia, especially if the patient takes multiple swallows for a single food bolus, or if the patient takes sips of water after each food bolus, or if the patient regurgitates food after swallowing [8].

8.1.4 Further Studies

Although the history and physical examination can provide numerous clues to arrive at possible diagnoses, additional tests are frequently needed, and the provider can tailor the workup to further evaluate the clinical suspicion.

In patients with suspected oropharyngeal disorders, the videofluoroscopic swallowing study is the gold standard for evaluating the swallowing mechanism [4, 5, 8, 12]. In this study, patients eat and drink foods that are mixed with barium to make them radiopaque. It is similar to the barium swallow, but the barium swallow specifies small food boluses and does not include drinking from a cup [4]. A videofluoroscopic swallowing study evaluates the anatomic structures, the movement of these structures, how food transits during swallowing, and how effective compensatory maneuvers (neck flexion or breath holding) are during swallowing. In this way, it is possible to develop an individualized diet by determining which food consistency is best and minimizes aspiration [4].

For patients with suspected esophageal dysphagia, providers may consider performing a barium swallow, upper endoscopy, or esophageal manometry. It is important to understand these studies are not identical or redundant; rather, they may provide complementary information. The decision on which study to perform first should be based on which test is most likely to yield the diagnosis and/or treat the pathology [4, 5, 8, 9, 12].

If the clinical picture is more consistent with esophageal motility dysfunction, a barium esophagram is the initial diagnostic test of choice. Barium esophagography allows for direct visualization of muscular function and coordination, evaluation of esophageal response to various food consistencies to replicate patients' symptoms, and evaluation of distal esophageal motility disorders including achalasia, scleroderma, or esophageal strictures, which are better evaluated by barium swallow as compared to endoscopy. Moreover, additional advantages of barium swallow are that it is noninvasive, is inexpensive, can be done in patients that are poor candidates for upper endoscopy, does not require sedation, has few complications, and can help plan future endoscopy, along with any associated procedures including botulinum injection or pneumatic dilatation. Barium studies are contraindicated in patients with suspected complete or near-complete obstruction, food impactions, and foreign body ingestions, for which endoscopy is diagnostic and therapeutic [2, 8, 9].

Upper endoscopy not only provides accurate information on esophageal anatomy, but it also allows for mucosal evaluation, the ability to biopsy, and the opportunity for therapeutic procedures if indicated [8]. By directly visualizing the gastrointestinal tract, endoscopy can diagnose intraluminal tumors, esophagitis, infection, food impaction, foreign body, and reflux disease, and it serves as a useful adjunct in the evaluation of motility disorders. Endoscopy is insensitive to diagnosing motility disorders, but contrary to barium esophagography, upper endoscopy has the opportunity for therapeutic potential either by pneumatic balloon dilatation, cautery, sclerotherapy, myotomy, or botulinum toxin injection [2, 9].

Esophageal manometry is presently the most sensitive technique and the gold standard in assessing and diagnosing esophageal motility disorders. Manometry, a diagnostic adjunct for patients with esophageal dysphagia, measures the peristaltic and sphincter function at intervals less than 1 cm apart along the entire esophagus [2, 4, 5, 8, 9, 12]. Recent evidence has demonstrated that the combination of manometry with impedance measurements is the most sensitive indicator of abnormal esophageal motility [8]. However, it is not a primary diagnostic study; rather, it is performed when a careful history, barium studies, and endoscopy have not elucidated a diagnosis [2].

The greatest concern in patients presenting with dysphagia is the possibility of having cancer as the cause of their symptoms. The evaluation of a patient who is suspected or confirmed to have esophageal cancer includes the previously mentioned studies, including upper endoscopy and endoscopic biopsy and barium esophagram. However, additional imaging is used to stage the cancer, including computed tomography to evaluate the mass and surrounding structures. Endoscopic ultrasound can identify adjacent nodal metastases and can direct needle biopsies of suspected nodal disease [9].

8.1.5 Management

The management of dysphagia depends on the etiology and typically involves medications and/or surgery (Table 8.3). Low-cost, low-risk, efficacious interventions include dietary modification with softer and smaller foods, behavioral or postural changes, and referral to a speech and language pathologist to strengthen oropharyngeal muscle groups. Careful monitoring of hydration, electrolytes, and nutrition is essential. Additional nutritional support may be warranted via parenteral or gastrostomy tube. Referral to specialist at an early stage may be indicated if the diagnosis remains unclear despite initial workup or if additional therapeutic expertise is required [2, 4, 5, 8].

Table 8.3 Treatment of common causes of dysphagia [2]

Achalasia—treated by reducing lower esophageal sphincter pressure by either pneumatic dilation or surgical myotomy. Pharmacologic therapy (botulinum toxin injection) may be used in patients with refractory symptoms or who are unwilling to undergo dilation or myotomy
Diffuse esophageal spasm and nutcracker esophagus—acid suppression with proton pump inhibitor (PPI), sublingual nitroglycerin, and calcium channel blockers. Botulinum toxin injection may reduce symptoms
Scleroderma and other autoimmune diseases are best treated with systemic management of the disease. Acid suppression with PPI is recommended
Rings, webs, and strictures are best managed with lifestyle and behavioral modifications. Acid suppression with PPI is recommended. With large lesions and refractory cases, endoscopic dilation, surgical resection, or electrocautery may be considered
Reflux esophagitis and Barrett's esophagus are best managed with lifestyle and behavioral modifications. Acid suppression with PPI or histamine-2 antagonists
Eosinophilic esophagitis should be managed by identifying allergic triggers via allergy testing and implementing aggressive diet modification to avoid those triggers. PPIs, swallowed topical steroids, and monoclonal antibody treatments are used as well [13]
Infectious esophagitis should be treated with the appropriate antiviral or antifungal agent. As infectious esophagitis is also commonly associated with immunosuppression, the disease should also be managed systemically
Esophageal carcinoma should be managed with chemotherapy, radiation, and/or surgery
Zenker's diverticulum can be managed via endoscopic cricopharyngeal myotomy

8.2 Odynophagia

It is important to distinguish dysphagia, which is the abnormal transit of solids and/or liquids, from odynophagia, which is pain during swallowing. As with dysphagia, odynophagia can be due to pain anywhere from the oropharynx to the esophagus. Odynophagia can also present alongside dysphagia, as the causes of dysphagia can also cause pain during swallowing.

8.2.1 Etiology

Pain during swallowing is due to inflammation of the gastrointestinal mucosa extending from the mouth to the distal esophagus. Inflammation can take the form of infection or local irritation. This topic will address the common causes of odynophagia and a brief summary of their treatments.

Common infectious causes include:

- Cytomegalovirus (CMV) esophagitis occurs exclusively in patients with immunocompromised states, such as posttransplantation, human immunodeficiency virus (HIV) infection or acquired immunodeficiency syndrome (AIDS), and long-term corticosteroid therapy. Because of the systemic effects of immunosuppression, CMV may present with symptoms involving secondary organ systems unrelated to the esophagus. Symptoms of CMV esophagitis may include nausea, vomiting, abdominal pain, odynophagia, dysphagia, weight loss, and retrosternal chest pain [14]. An induction course of intravenous antivirals such as ganciclovir is necessary before a patient can be maintained on an oral regimen of valganciclovir [15].

- Herpes simplex virus (HSV) esophagitis is commonly seen in immunocompromised patients, such as posttransplantation, corticosteroid therapy, HIV and AIDS, and post-chemotherapy, but can also be seen in immunocompetent individuals [15]. Symptoms include retrosternal chest pain, odynophagia, dysphagia, fever, weight loss, nausea, vomiting, and food impaction. Case reports have described gastrointestinal bleeding and the development of tracheoesophageal fistulae as possible sequela of HSV esophagitis due to the ulcerations that occur [16–19]. Immunocompetent individuals may not require treatment but can be treated with short courses of oral acyclovir. Immunosuppressed patients require longer courses of treatment. Patients not tolerating oral medications due to dysphagia or odynophagia may require admission for parenteral antivirals [15].
- Candidiasis (thrush) is an opportunistic infection commonly seen in immunocompromised states. Patients with HIV who are not on highly active antiretroviral therapy (HAART) or who are on HAART but have not achieved immune reconstitution are at particular risk for candidiasis. The absence of oropharyngeal candidiasis does not rule out candidal esophagitis. However, the presence of oropharyngeal candidiasis carries a positive predictive value of 90% for esophageal candidiasis [20]. One- to two-week courses of oral antifungal medications are used to treat candidal esophagitis. Some patients with recurrent episodes require prophylactic daily antifungals. Oral candidiasis often only requires topical antifungals [15].
- Pharyngitis is a common source of infection that causes sore throat and odynophagia and may be caused by viral (influenza, CMV, EBV, HSV, HIV) or bacterial causes. Group A streptococcus is the most common bacterial cause, although other groups of streptococcus, *Corynebacterium diphtheriae*, *Mycoplasma pneumoniae*, and others can cause pharyngitis as well. The differential diagnosis for viral or bacterial pharyngitis should include consideration of emergent conditions, including epiglottitis, peritonsillar abscess, retropharyngeal abscess, and submandibular deep tissue infections. These conditions typically present with copious secretions, dysphonia, drooling, muffled "hot potato" voice, hoarseness, trismus, and neck or submandibular swelling. The clinician should have a high level of suspicion for these infections; if there is any suspicion, the patient should be emergently transferred to the emergency department for definitive care.
- Aphthous ulcers are recurrent, round, small, painful ulcers located in the oropharynx and usually last less than 2 weeks. The cause of these ulcers is poorly understood [21]. Topical anesthetics are the mainstay of treatment, as well as avoiding irritating foods and beverages.
- Gingivostomatitis primarily affects children and their close contacts and causes clusters of small, painful oral ulcerations. Parents of affected children may notice the lesions, or they may express concerns of fever, decreased oral intake, or fussiness in small children. Subtypes include hand, foot, and mouth disease, herpangina, and herpetic gingivostomatitis. Hand, foot, and mouth disease is highly contagious and caused by specific strains of coxsackievirus. It primarily affects

children but has been reported in adults who are in close contact with infected individuals [22]. Patients and parents should be educated on hand hygiene to prevent spread of infection to close contacts. Children in particular should be evaluated for signs of dehydration and given topical and systemic analgesics to facilitate their oral intake [22].

Causes of local irritation include:

- Esophageal foreign bodies may cause retrosternal chest pain, dysphagia, globus sensation, drooling, stridor, wheezing, or choking. High-risk foreign bodies (e.g., sharp objects, batteries, magnets) or foreign bodies that have been present for extended periods of time can cause esophageal erosion, resulting in esophageal perforation. Perforation can result in pneumomediastinum and mediastinitis due to contamination of the mediastinum with gastrointestinal flora. A patient with esophageal perforation may be toxic- or ill-appearing with signs of sepsis such as fever and tachycardia, respiratory distress, or crepitus (i.e., Hamman's crunch). These patients should be emergently transferred to an emergency department for stabilization and gastroenterology and thoracic surgery consultation [23].
- Local trauma to the esophagus can result from diagnostic investigations (e.g., endoscopy), drinking hot foods/drinks, ingesting caustic substances, reflux, or localized radiation in the treatment of cancer. Localized trauma can cause mucosal irritation and subsequent fibrosis, resulting in not only odynophagia but also dysphagia.

References

1. Speyer R, et al. White paper by the European Society for Swallowing Disorders: screening and non-instrumental assessment for dysphagia in adults. Dysphagia. 2022;37(2):333–49.
2. Kruger D. Assessing esophageal dysphagia. JAAPA. 2014;27(5):23–30.
3. Clavé P, Shaker R. Dysphagia: current reality and scope of the problem. Nat Rev Gastroenterol Hepatol. 2015;12(5):259–70.
4. Palmer JB, Drennan JC, Baba M. Evaluation and treatment of swallowing impairments. Am Fam Physician. 2000;61(8):2453–62.
5. American Gastroenterological Association. American Gastroenterological Association medical position statement on management of oropharyngeal dysphagia. Gastroenterology. 1999;116(2):452–4.
6. Panara K, Ahangar ER, Padali D. Physiology, swallowing. In: StatPearls [Internet]. Treasure Island (FL): StatPearls Publishing; 2021.
7. Malone JC, Arya NR. Anatomy, head and neck, swallowing. In: StatPearls [Internet]. Treasure Island (FL): StatPearls Publishing; 2021.
8. Abdel Jalil AA, Katzka DA, Castell DO. Approach to the patient with dysphagia. Am J Med. 2015;128(10):1138.e17–23.
9. Navaneethan U, Eubanks S. Approach to patients with esophageal dysphagia. Surg Clin N Am. 2015;95(3):483–9.

10. Hendrix TR. Art and science of history taking in the patient with difficulty swallowing. Dysphagia. 1993;8(2):69–73.
11. Krill JT, Naik RD, Vaezi MF. Clinical management of achalasia: current state of the art. Clin Exp Gastroenterol. 2016;9:71–82.
12. Lind CD. Dysphagia: evaluation and treatment. Gastroenterol Clin N Am. 2003;32(2):553–75.
13. Biedermann L, et al. Eosinophilic esophagitis-established facts and new horizons. Semin Immunopathol. 2021;43(3):319–35.
14. Wilcox CM, Straub RF, Schwartz DA. Prospective evaluation of biopsy number for the diagnosis of viral esophagitis in patients with HIV infection and esophageal ulcer. Gastrointest Endosc. 1996;44(5):587–93.
15. Rosołowski M, Kierzkiewicz M. Etiology, diagnosis and treatment of infectious esophagitis. Prz Gastroenterol. 2013;8(6):333–7.
16. Rattner HM, Cooper DJ, Zaman MB. Severe bleeding from herpes esophagitis. Am J Gastroenterol. 1985;80(7):523–5.
17. Cirillo NW, Lyon DT, Schuller AM. Tracheoesophageal fistula complicating herpes esophagitis in AIDS. Am J Gastroenterol. 1993;88(4):587–9.
18. Obrecht WF, et al. Tracheoesophageal fistula: a serious complication of infectious esophagitis. Gastroenterology. 1984;87(5):1174–9.
19. Marshall JB, et al. Herpes esophagitis causing an unsuspected esophageal food bolus impaction in an institutionalized patient. J Clin Gastroenterol. 1992;15(2):179–80.
20. Wilcox CM, Straub RF, Clark WS. Prospective evaluation of oropharyngeal findings in human immunodeficiency virus-infected patients with esophageal ulceration. Am J Gastroenterol. 1995;90(11):1938–41.
21. Ship JA. Recurrent aphthous stomatitis. An update. Oral Surg Oral Med Oral Pathol Oral Radiol Endod. 1996;81(2):141–7.
22. Repass GL, Palmer WC, Stancampiano FF. Hand, foot, and mouth disease: identifying and managing an acute viral syndrome. Cleve Clin J Med. 2014;81(9):537–43.
23. DeVivo A, et al. High risk and low prevalence diseases: esophageal perforation. Am J Emerg Med. 2022;53:29–36.

Noncardiac Chest Pain (Including Chest Wall Pain) 9

Dipal Shah

9.1 Introduction

Chest pain is of particular interest to emergency physicians, both for its high prevalence and its potential to reflect serious disease. Each year, 7.6 million Americans seek emergency department care for chest pain, representing 5% of all visits and the second most common presenting symptom overall [1].

Emergency physicians are perhaps most attuned to evaluating for cardiac causes of chest pain. Heart disease is the leading cause of death in the United States, and 1–4% of patients presenting to the ED with chest pain are suffering an acute coronary syndrome or myocardial infarction [2, 3].

All chest pain investigations should at least consider the possibility of cardiac diseases as a cause. These include coronary artery disease, unstable angina, myocardial infarction, congestive heart failure, valvular disease, and aortic dissection. Several predictive tools are available to help risk stratify the likelihood of acute coronary conditions [4]. Potentially life-threatening noncardiac causes, including pneumothorax and pulmonary embolism, should also be considered.

Nevertheless, most chest pain is not life-threatening or cardiac in origin. In one meta-analysis, only 14–16% of chest pain was cardiac [3]. In comparison, 25–50% was musculoskeletal, 10–18% pulmonary, 6–10% gastrointestinal, and 10–18% psychogenic. Recurrent noncardiac chest pain is especially common, affecting approximately one in four American adults [5]. Patients suffering from such pain are more likely to report a diminished quality of life and higher rates of depression and anxiety [6]. Thus, care must be given to investigate and treat noncardiac causes as well.

D. Shah (✉)
University of Central Florida, Orlando, FL, USA

B. K. Desai et al. (eds.), *Primary Care for Emergency Physicians*,
https://doi.org/10.1007/978-3-031-64676-8_9

9.2 Risk Factors for Chest Pain

Compared to patients with cardiac chest pain, patients with noncardiac chest pain are younger, smoke more tobacco, drink more alcohol, and have higher rates of anxiety [5].

- Hypertension
- Hyperlipidemia
- Tobacco use
- Alcohol use
- Diabetes
- Coronary artery disease
- Family history of coronary artery disease
- Increasing age
  - Likelihood of noncardiac chest pain decreases with age
  - Likelihood of cardiac chest pain increases with age
- Sedentary lifestyle
- Obesity
- Heartburn
- Acid reflux
- Dysphagia
- Emotional stress
- Depression
- Anxiety

9.3 Differential Diagnosis

- Cardiac chest pain
  - Ischemic
    - Stable angina
    - Unstable angina
    - Myocardial infarction
    - Congestive heart failure
  - Nonischemic
    - Pericarditis
    - Myocarditis
    - Cardiac tamponade
    - Valvular heart disease
    - Aortic dissection
- Noncardiac chest pain
  - Gastroesophageal
    - Gastroesophageal reflux disease (GERD)
    - Peptic ulcer disease
    - Gastritis and esophagitis

    - Esophageal spasm
    - Esophageal dysmotility
    - Esophageal rupture
    - Hiatal hernia
    - Pancreatitis
  - Pulmonary
    - Pneumonia
    - Bronchitis
    - Tracheitis
    - Lung disease
      - COPD
      - Asthma
      - Restrictive lung disease
    - Lung cancer
      - Chest pain is a presenting symptom in 53% [7]
    - Pneumothorax
    - Pulmonary embolism
    - Pleuritis
  - Musculoskeletal
    - Costochondritis
    - Tietze syndrome
    - Chest wall syndromes
    - Overuse injuries
    - Trauma
      - Rib fractures or contusions
      - Thoracic spinal fractures
      - Sternal fractures
    - Skin and soft tissue
      - Breast lesions
      - Herpes zoster
  - Psychiatric
    - Emotional stress
    - Hyperventilation
    - Anxiety disorders
    - Panic disorders
    - Somatoform disorders

Red Flags of Chest Pain

- Cardiac chest pain red flags
  - Signs of cardiac ischemia or infarction
    - Exertional chest pain
    - Pain radiating to the arm, shoulder, neck, or jaw
    - Nausea
    - Diaphoresis

    - New EKG changes
      - ST segment elevations
      - ST segment depressions
      - T wave inversions
      - Hyperacute T waves
      - Q waves
      - Conduction deficits
  - Murmur
  - Friction rub
  - Abnormal rhythm
  - Pulmonary edema
  - Sudden onset of acute ripping or tearing pain
    - May suggest aortic dissection
    - Incidence is six cases per 100,000 patient years [7]
- Noncardiac chest pain red flags
  - Gastrointestinal
    - Repeated vomiting
    - Decreased appetite
    - Unintentional weight loss
    - Dysphagia or odynophagia
    - Hematemesis
    - Melena
  - Pulmonary
    - Acute, pleuritic chest pain with dyspnea, tachypnea, tachycardia, or hypoxia
      - Suggests pneumothorax
        - Acute pleuritic pain with dyspnea is present in 64–85% of pneumothorax cases [7]
    - Dyspnea, tachycardia, clear lung sounds, cough, hemoptysis, or signs of deep vein thrombosis (unilateral limb swelling)
      - Suggests pulmonary embolism (PE)
      - Wells score less than 2 and normal D-dimer assay excludes PE
      - Patients with elevated Wells score or D-dimer may require CT angiography or ventilation-perfusion scan
    - Cough, sputum, fever, and tachypnea with signs of severe sepsis or septic shock
      - Suggests pneumonia with concerning features
    - Dyspnea, hoarseness, cough, hemoptysis, and unintentional weight loss, especially in a smoker
      - May suggest lung cancer
  - Musculoskeletal
    - Severe mechanism
    - Poor air movement secondary to pain
  - Psychiatric
    - Suicidal thoughts

Thoughts of self-harm

9.4 History

History is directed at detecting red flag symptoms and eliciting information that may clarify the timing, chronicity, severity, and source of the patient's chest pain.

Important historical features to elicit include:

- Characteristics of chest pain
  - Onset
  - Duration
    Acute vs. chronic
  - Quality
  - Severity
  - Time course
  - Location
  - Radiation
  - Possible inciting factors
  - Alleviating and aggravating factors
- Other acute medical complaints
  - Dyspnea
  - Palpitations
  - Diaphoresis
  - Cough or sputum
  - Wheezing
  - Fever
  - Heartburn
  - Nausea or vomiting
  - Weight loss
  - Anxiety
- Past medical history
- Family history (especially of early myocardial infarctions)
- Use of medications or drugs (including caffeine, alcohol, tobacco, cocaine, and supplements)
- Psychiatric history

9.5 Physical Examination

The physical examination should focus on potential emergency conditions.

- Vital sign assessment
  - Fever or hypothermia may suggest an infectious etiology
  - Hypoxia may indicate a pulmonary or vascular etiology

  - Tachycardia
  - Pulse oximetry can detect hypoxia
- Cardiovascular assessment should focus on:
  - Heart sounds
  - Regular or irregular rhythm
  - Murmurs, friction rub, or gallop rhythms
  - Jugular venous distention (JVD)
  - Peripheral edema or swelling
  - Pulse differential in the upper extremities
- Pulmonary assessment should focus on:
  - Cyanosis
  - Lung sounds
    - Crackles
    - Wheezes
    - Rhonchi
    - Stridor
    - Egophony
  - Dullness to percussion
  - Unilateral absence or decrease of lung sounds
    - May suggest pneumothorax
  - Reproducible pain
- Musculoskeletal assessment should focus on:
  - Localized tenderness
  - Swelling
  - Skin lesions
  - Reproducible pain
- Gastrointestinal assessment should focus on:
  - Epigastric tenderness
  - Vomiting
  - Heme-positive stool (if pertinent)
  - Signs of anemia
- Psychiatric assessment should focus on:
  - Hyperventilation
  - Suicidal thoughts
  - Thoughts of self-harm
  - Anxiety or panic states

9.6 Introduction to Treatment

After evaluation and stabilization of emergency conditions, the emergency physician has several options to treat chest pain. These include:

1. Education and lifestyle modification
   (a) Tobacco and alcohol cessation

   (b) Avoidance of caffeine, stimulants, and fresh citrus juice
   (c) Minimization of opioids and benzodiazepines
   (d) Home medication compliance
   (e) Exercise and dietary modifications
   (f) Stress reduction techniques
2. Medications
   (a) Analgesics for pain relief
      (A) Aspirin
      (B) Nonsteroidal anti-inflammatory drugs (NSAIDs)
      (C) Opioids
   (b) Anti-inflammatory medications
      (A) Nonsteroidal anti-inflammatory drugs (NSAIDs).
      (B) Aspirin
   (c) Anti-reflux medications for gastrointestinal pain
      (A) Proton pump inhibitors (PPIs)
      (B) H2 receptor antagonists
   (d) Antibiotics for infections (e.g., pneumonia)
   (e) Psychiatric medications for anxiety, depression, or pain modulation
      (A) Includes benzodiazepines and antidepressants
      (B) Many emergency physicians will defer initiation of psychiatric medications to a psychiatrist or primary care physician
3. Referral and follow-up
   (a) Primary care physician
   (b) Cardiology for suspected coronary artery disease
   (c) Gastroenterology
      (A) Lifestyle modifications
      (B) Upper endoscopy
      (C) Esophageal manometry
      (D) Empiric PPI trial
      (E) Muscle relaxant trial
      (F) Pain modulators
      (G) Botulinum toxin
      (H) Surgical or endoscopic therapy
   (d) Psychiatry or psychology

9.7 Pharmacologic Treatment

9.7.1 Nonsteroidal Anti-inflammatory Drugs (NSAIDs)

Provide immediate pain relief and anti-inflammatory effect.

Side effects of these medications include gastrointestinal ulcers, bleeding, and acute kidney injury.

Examples of NSAIDs
Aspirin
Ibuprofen
Naproxen
Ketorolac
Meloxicam
Indomethacin
Ketoprofen

Pitfalls

1. Prescribing to patients at risk for bleeding
2. Prescribing to patients with kidney disease
3. Prescribing long-term doses
4. Failing to suggest to take with food

9.7.2 Opioid Analgesics

Provide potent and immediate pain relief.

Side effects of these medications include nausea, lightheadedness, and fatigue.

Examples of opioids
Codeine
Fentanyl
Hydrocodone
Morphine
Oxycodone

Pitfalls

1. Sedation
2. Respiratory depression and apnea
3. No anti-inflammatory effect
4. Constipation
5. Dependence, addiction, and withdrawal
6. Risk of overdose

9.7.3 Proton Pump Inhibitors (PPIs)

Provide long-lasting reduction of gastric acid production.

GERD is present in up to 60% of patients with noncardiac chest pain [8]. Acid reflux causes symptoms of heartburn in some patients and chest pain in others. In patients with suspicion of GERD and frequent symptoms impairing quality of life, gastroenterologists recommend that a proton pump inhibitor (PPI) be initiated at a high dose and tapered to the lowest dose that maintains symptomatic relief. Along with lifestyle modifications, this technique has a high success rate [5].

Examples of proton pump inhibitors (PPIs)
Esomeprazole
Lansoprazole
Omeprazole
Pantoprazole
Rabeprazole

Pitfalls

1. Failure to taper dose once relief is achieved
2. Some studies show an association between PPIs and diarrheal infection or pneumonia

9.7.4 H2 Receptor Antagonists (H2 Blockers)

Provide long-lasting reduction of gastric acid production.

H2 blockers are less effective than PPIs in reducing GERD-related noncardiac chest pain; however, they may be used in patients with minimal symptoms as initial treatment [5]. They successfully control the symptoms of GERD-related noncardiac chest pain in 42–52% of patients [9].

Examples of H2 receptor antagonists
Cimetidine
Famotidine
Ranitidine

Pitfalls

1. Generally well tolerated
2. Some studies show an association between PPIs and diarrheal infection or pneumonia

9.7.5 Benzodiazepines

These are a class of psychoactive medications producing immediate short-term relief of anxiety or panic disorder.

A short course of this class of medication may be considered in consultation with the patient's primary care physician or psychiatrist.

Examples of benzodiazepines
Alprazolam Chlordiazepoxide Clonazepam Diazepam Lorazepam

Pitfalls

1. Respiratory depression or apnea
2. Sedation
3. Dependence, addiction, and withdrawal
4. Risk of overdose

9.7.6 Antidepressants

These medications can help with long-term management of various psychiatric conditions.

A short course of this class of medication may be considered in consultation with the patient's primary care physician or psychiatrist.

Examples of antidepressants
Amitriptyline Bupropion Citalopram Duloxetine Escitalopram Fluoxetine Paroxetine Sertraline Venlafaxine

Pitfalls

1. Use in pregnancy
2. Anticholinergic effects
3. Sedation
4. Weight changes
5. Sexual dysfunction
6. May paradoxically increase risk of suicide

References

1. National Hospital Ambulatory Medical Care Survey. 2017. Emergency department summary tables. https://www.cdc.gov/nchs/data/nhamcs/web_tables/2017_ed_web_tables-508.pdf.
2. Ebell MH. Evaluation of chest pain in primary care patients Am Fam Physician. 2011;83(5):603–5.
3. Haasenritter J, Biroga T, Keunecke C, et al. Causes of chest pain in primary care—a systematic review and meta-analysis. Croat Med J. 2010;56(5):422–30.
4. Ayerbe L, González E, Gallo V, et al. Clinical assessment of patients with chest pain; a systematic review of predictive tools. BMC Cardiovasc Disord. 2016;6(1):18.
5. Schey R, Villarreal A, Fass R. Noncardiac chest pain: current treatment. Gastroenterol Hepatol. 2007;3(4):255–62.
6. Eslick GD, Jones MP, Talley NJ. Non-cardiac chest pain: prevalence, risk factors, impact and consulting—a population-based study. Aliment Pharmacol Ther. 2003;17(9):1115–24.
7. Yelland M, Cayley WE Jr, Vach W. An algorithm for the diagnosis and management of chest pain in primary care. Med Clin N Am. 2010;94(2):349–74.
8. Liuzzo JP, Ambrose JA. Chest pain from gastroesophageal reflux disease in patients with coronary artery disease. Cardiol Rev. 2005;13:167–73.
9. Fang J, Bjorkman D. A critical approach to noncardiac chest pain: pathophysiology, diagnosis, and treatment. Am J Gastroenterol. 2001;96:958–68.

Hypertension in the Emergency Department

10

James Medley

10.1 Introduction

Hypertension is one of the most common conditions seen in primary care with complications including myocardial infarction, heart failure [1], stroke, chronic kidney disease, and death if not detected early and treated appropriately [2]. Abundant evidence has shown benefit of antihypertensive treatment in reducing important health outcomes in persons with hypertension [2].

Even then, most asymptomatic patients with poorly controlled hypertension do not have acute target organ damage and thus do not require immediate workup or treatment. When a patient presents with severely elevated blood pressure (BP), the emergency physician's need to differentiate hypertensive emergency (requiring investigation, treatment, and probable admission) from simple uncontrolled hypertension (requiring close primary care follow-up and possibly a bridge prescription to begin antihypertensive treatment).

10.2 Definitions

10.2.1 Hypertension

The American College of Cardiology and the American Heart Association (ACC/AHA) updated the definition of hypertension in a 2017 statement [3].

- Normal: systolic blood pressure (SBP) <120 mmHg *and* diastolic blood pressure (DBP) <80 mmHg

J. Medley (✉)
Department of Community Health and Family Medicine, University of Florida College of Medicine, Gainesville, FL, USA
e-mail: jmed617@ufl.edu

B. K. Desai et al. (eds.), *Primary Care for Emergency Physicians*,
https://doi.org/10.1007/978-3-031-64676-8_10

- Elevated blood pressure: SBP 120 mmHg to 129 *and* DBP <80 mmHg
- Stage 1 hypertension: SBP 130–139 mmHg *or* DBP 80–89 mmHg
- Stage 2 hypertension: SBP ≥140 mmHg *or* DBP ≥90 mmHg

Isolated systolic or diastolic blood pressure can be described when only one value falls into the hypertensive range, while the other value stays within the normal or elevated range.

Note that these values rely on measurement using proper technique, and elevated values should be confirmed with measurements taken with proper technique [3].

Proper technique for blood pressure measurement includes the following [4]:

- The patient has been seated comfortably for 5 min in a quiet environment
- Feet flat on the floor with legs and ankles uncrossed
- Arm resting at heart level
- Greater than 30 min since caffeine intake, tobacco use, or exercise [5].

Diagnosis of hypertension typically requires more than one value in the hypertensive range, in optimal conditions, or other forms of measurement such as home readings or ambulatory monitoring [3]. This author posits that in the absence of a known hypertension diagnosis or definite hypertensive urgency/emergency (discussed below), a diagnosis of "elevated blood pressure" will suffice, and primary care follow-up should be arranged.

10.2.2 Severe Hypertension, Urgency, and Emergency

There is no universal set limit for severe hypertension in adults. Severe hypertension in adults is often defined as SBP ≥180 mmHg or DBP ≥110–120 mmHg in the literature [6, 7].

Other terms such as hypertensive urgency, hypertensive crisis, etc., have been used in the literature with some ambiguity. Rosen's emergency medicine textbook suggests a more practical classification for management of hypertension at the ED [5]:

- **Hypertensive emergency**
  - Significantly elevated BP with signs or symptoms of acute, ongoing target organ damage [8] which may include:

    Neurologic: hypertensive encephalopathy and hemorrhagic/ischemic cerebral vascular accident

    Cardiovascular: myocardial ischemia or infarction, acute heart failure, acute pulmonary edema, arterial dissection, and unstable angina pectoris

    Others: acute renal failure/insufficiency, hypertensive retinopathy, eclampsia, and microangiopathic hemolytic anemia [9]

- **Hypertensive urgency**
  - Also referred to as severe asymptomatic hypertension
  - Includes significant BP elevation without symptoms or signs of target organ damage

    Still requires evaluation, including possible workup such as EKG, renal function monitoring, etc., to ensure no evidence of target organ damage

10.3 Etiology and Risk Factors

Non-modifiable

- Genetics (twice as much risk if one or two parents are hypertensive) [10, 11].
- Age (advanced age associated with increased risk).
- Gender (male > female).
- Reduced adult nephron mass may predispose to hypertension, which may be genetic or acquired (hypoxia, drugs, nutritional deficiency), due to premature birth, or infection.

Modifiable

- Being overweight
- High-sodium diet
- Excessive alcohol intake
- Sedentary lifestyle (defined as less than 150 min of moderately intense exercise weekly)
- High stress
- Smoking
- Diabetes
- Hyperlipidemia
- Personality traits and depression

10.4 Differential Diagnosis of Underlying Causes [12]

Cardiovascular

- Primary hypertension
- Acute coronary syndrome
- Aortic dissection
- Coarctation of aorta
- Vasculitis
- Heart failure
- Collagen vascular disease

Renal

- Acute or chronic renal failure
- Glomerulonephritis
- Renal artery stenosis

Endocrine/electrolytes

- Pheochromocytoma
- Cushing's syndrome (including iatrogenic hypercortisolism)
- Hyperestrogenism, including contraceptive agent use
- Hyperthyroidism
- Primary aldosteronism
- Congenital adrenal hyperplasia
- Acromegaly
- Hypercalcemia

Respiratory

- Obstructive sleep apnea
- Respiratory distress

Psych/CNS

- Anxiety
- White coat syndrome
- Acute cerebrovascular accident
- Intracranial mass
- Acute or severe pain
- Bulbar poliomyelitis
- Intracranial hypertension

Obstetrics

- Gestational hypertension
- Preeclampsia or eclampsia

Drug/medication related

- Rebound hypertension (discontinuation effect from antihypertensives especially beta-adrenergic antagonists)
- Over-the-counter medications
  - NSAIDs and stimulant decongestants
- Immunosuppressants
  - Cyclosporine and tacrolimus

- Recreational sympathomimetic drugs
  - Cocaine, amphetamines, phencyclidine, etc.
- Herbal supplements
  - St. John's Wort
- Industrial chemicals
  - Lead, mercury, thallium, and lithium salts
- Alcohol withdrawal
- Antipsychotics, antidepressants, and anxiolytics (venlafaxine, buspirone, etc.)
- Serotonin syndrome
- Weight loss stimulants (e.g., phentermine)
- Erythropoietin
- Metoclopramide
- Ketamine

10.5 History

ED physicians should always be vigilant in diagnosing acute, ongoing, target organ damage in hypertensive emergency. A history including the following can be invaluable in this endeavor [13]:

- Recent head trauma.
- Generalized neurologic symptoms:
  - Mental status alteration.
  - Agitation.
  - Delirium.
  - Seizure.
- Nausea and vomiting:
  - Suspect increased intracranial pressure or toxin ingestion.
- Focal neurologic symptoms:
  - Consider cerebrovascular accident, intracranial mass, or increased intracranial pressure.
- Chest discomfort:
  - May be a sign of myocardial ischemia or aortic dissection.
- Dyspnea:
  - May be a sign of pulmonary edema.
  - May be a sign of pulmonary embolism.
- Acute, severe back pain:
  - May be a sign of aortic dissection.
- Pregnancy:
  - Preeclampsia.
  - Increased risk of aortic dissection in pregnancy.
- Sympathomimetic drugs:
  - Cocaine.
  - Amphetamine(s).

  - Phencyclidine.
  - Monoamine oxidase inhibitors.
- Recent discontinuation of sympatholytic agents.
- Include a medication review.
- Social history can be an important indicator of exposures, diet, exercise, and stress.

10.6 Physical Exam

Ensure an accurate BP reading as much as possible, including rechecking any outlying readings. Recall the goal of the physical exam is both to attempt evaluation for hypertensive emergency (the prime directive of the emergency physician) and also to discover a potential cause of secondary hypertension.

Important aspects of the physical examination include [14]:

- General appearance
  - Distribution of body fat
  - Skin lesions
  - Muscle strength
  - Alertness
- Fundoscopy especially with vision changes
  - Hemorrhage
  - Papilledema
  - Cotton wool spots
- Neck
  - Palpation and auscultation of carotids
  - Thyroid
- Heart
  - Size (displaced PMI)
  - Rhythm
  - Sounds
- Lungs
  - Rhonchi
  - Rales
- Abdomen
  - Renal masses
  - Bruits over aorta or renal arteries
  - Femoral pulses
- Extremities
  - Peripheral pulses
  - Edema
- Neurologic assessment
  - Visual disturbance
  - Focal weakness
  - Confusion

10.7 Diagnostic Testing

There is no consensus about the necessary laboratory workup of patients with severe asymptomatic hypertension or hypertension significantly over baseline, but recommendations focus on identifying underlying complications that may be clinically silent and to identify medical conditions that may further direct antihypertensive therapy [8, 13]. In symptomatic patients, a similar testing battery may be reasonable still, though symptoms and physical exam abnormalities will certainly direct testing more precisely.

Testing for target organ injury may include EKG, cardiac troponin, chest radiography especially if lung exam is limited or unreliable, pregnancy testing, serum electrolytes and creatinine, and head imaging if hemorrhage may be suspected. TSH can be considered if evaluation is consistent with a hyperthyroid state

10.8 Treatment and Disposition of Patients with Hypertension

10.8.1 Asymptomatic Hypertension

Managing asymptomatic hypertension at the ED is different from the primary care setting. Rapidly lowering BP in the ED is usually unnecessary in asymptomatic patients and may be harmful. In most cases, no intervention is necessary, and an outpatient follow-up should be scheduled with the primary care provider within the next month, preferably within the next few days after the emergency encounter.

Lifestyle modification is recommended for all patients with hypertension, including salt reduction, counseling regarding the DASH diet and physical activity, smoking cessation, and alcohol moderation [15, 16]. While lifestyle counseling in a busy emergency department may not be feasible, providing handouts or briefly discussing lifestyle topics may help the patient to engage with his or her primary care provider at the follow-up visit.

10.8.2 Hypertensive Urgency [17]

In the absence of hypertensive urgency, asymptomatic severe hypertension typically requires treatment within the emergency setting with close outpatient follow-up. In general, the blood pressure should be lowered to <160 SBP and <100 DBP in this time frame.

In general, it is recommended to avoid lowering the mean arterial pressure (MAP) more than 30% acutely, so discharging a patient with blood pressures above those recommendations may be required if their initial presenting pressures were very high.

There is no present high-quality evidence guiding the decision on timing of blood pressure reduction, without proven benefit from rapid lowering of blood pressure in these patients. The clinical decision on blood pressure reduction timing depends on:

1. The risk of complications from rapid lowering of blood pressure including stroke (hypoperfusion in significant cerebrovascular disease), myocardial infarction, and acute kidney injury (both prerenal decreased effective circulating volume and acute ischemic tubular necrosis).
2. The risk of secondary complications developing from continued elevations in blood pressure.

In all patients, a quiet room can have a significant effect in blood pressure, with decreases in 20+ mmHg SBP and 10+ mmHg DBP observed in one study after 30 min in a quiet area [18].

For patients who may require rapid (i.e., over hours) blood pressure improvements, oral clonidine and oral captopril are reasonable choices as they have faster onset of action. It should be noted that clonidine is not a preferred long-term agent so patient counseling may be helpful to improve expectations that this may be changed at the follow-up visit. In addition, volume-overloaded patients should avoid captopril and may benefit from other therapy [17].

Otherwise, resuming the patient's standard antihypertensive regimen is a reasonable option especially if lack of access to these medications contributed to high values. This author recommends exploring the root causes to medication interruption to avoid placing the patient in the same situation in the near future.

If the emergency physician is starting a new blood pressure medication for the patient, there is no consistent evidence that any one agent is the ideal first-line medication. Certainly, taking comorbidities into account can be helpful (e.g., angiotensin-converting enzyme inhibitors or angiotensin receptor blockers for patients with diabetes mellitus or a thiazide diuretic for patients with heart failure). Additionally, side effect profiles can help eliminate agents from consideration (e.g., beta-adrenergic antagonists should be used with caution in patients with diabetes mellitus or asthma, and diuretics used with caution in those at risk for dehydration).

Initial antihypertensive treatment could include [3]:

- In general nonblack population:
  - A thiazide diuretic, calcium channel blocker (CCB), angiotensin-converting enzyme (ACE) inhibitor, or angiotensin II receptor blockers (ARB) alone or in combination.
- In the general black population:
  - A thiazide diuretic or CCB alone or in combination.

    Note: the current best evidence suggests decreased efficacy of ACE inhibitors or ARBs alone in black patients, though further investigation of this trend may be needed to ensure no bias exists in these studies.
- In patients with chronic kidney disease older than 18 years old:
  - ACE inhibitor or ARBs alone or in combination with other drug classes.

- In patients with heart failure:
  - Thiazide diuretics, ACE inhibitors, and CCBs are more effective respectively.
- In general, the JNC 8 report does not recommend α-blockers or β-blockers for the initial treatment of hypertension.

Note that ACE inhibitors and ARBs cannot be used concurrently and both are contraindicated in pregnancy.

A more detailed discussion of specific medications is included below:

10.8.3 Evidence-Based Dosing for Antihypertensive Drugs*

ACE inhibitors:

Medication	Initial daily dose (mg)	Target dose (mg)	Doses/day
Captopril	50	150–200	2
Enalapril	5	20	1–2
Lisinopril	10	40	1

Pitfalls:

- Contraindicated in pregnancy. Caution in women of childbearing age
- May cause a chronic cough
- May cause life-threatening angioedema of head and neck (this author suggests initiating antihypertensive therapy with ARBs rather than ACE inhibitors as they carry the same benefits with a much lower risk of angioedema)
- Avoid in bilateral renal stenosis
- May predispose to hyperkalemia
- May cause increase in serum creatinine

Angiotensin receptor blockers (ARBs)

Medication	Initial daily dose, mg	Target dose, mg	No. of doses/day
Candesartan	4	12–32	1
Losartan	50	100	1–2
Valsartan	40–80	160–320	1

Pitfalls:

- Contraindicated in pregnancy. Caution in women of childbearing age
- Avoid in bilateral renal stenosis
- May cause angioedema, though risk is significantly less than with ACE inhibitors
- May predispose to hyperkalemia
- May cause increase in serum creatinine

β-Blockers

Medication	Initial daily dose, mg	Target dose, mg	No. of doses/day
Atenolol	25–50	100	1
Metoprolol	50	100–200	1–2

Pitfalls:

- Abrupt stopping may cause tachyarrhythmia and potential cardiac ischemia.
- JNC 8 does not recommend β-blockers for the initial treatment of hypertension.
- Bronchospasm in asthma or COPD (nonselective agents).
- May delay symptoms of hypoglycemia in patients with diabetes mellitus.

Calcium channel blockers

Medication	Initial daily dose, mg	Target dose, mg	No. of doses/day
Amlodipine	2.5	10	1
Diltiazem XR	120–180	360	1
Nitrendipine	10	20	1–2

Pitfalls:

- May cause second- and third-degree heart block, left ventricular dysfunction (except amlodipine)
- May cause peripheral edema

Thiazide-type diuretics

Medication	Initial daily dose, mg	Target dose, mg	No. of doses/day
Chlorthalidone	12.5	12.5–25	1
Hydrochlorothiazide	12.5–25	25–50	1–2
Indapamide	1.25	1.25–2.5	1

Pitfalls:

- May cause electrolyte imbalance (hypokalemia, hyponatremia, hypercalcemia).
- Caution in patients with gout.
- Check BUN/Cr and electrolytes at baseline and make sure patient follows up.
- Usually ineffective with CrCl <30 mL/min unless in combination with a loop diuretic.

**The above mentioned list and dosing is adopted from JNC8 based on the randomized clinical trials reviewed by JNC8 and does not include other drug classes that are not recommended as first-line therapy* [1]

Many people will require treatment with more than one antihypertensive drug to achieve BP control. JNC8 suggests that any of the four classes (ACE inhibitors,

ARB, CCB, and thiazide diuretics) would be good choices as add-on agents. Also the JNC8 recommendation is specific for thiazide-type diuretics and does not include loop or potassium-sparing diuretics [1]

10.9 Hypertensive Emergency

In hypertensive emergencies, the BP should be aggressively lowered within minutes to an hour by no more than 25% and then lowered to 160/100–110 mm Hg within the next 2–6 h [13]. It is beyond the scope of this chapter to discuss treatment of this true medical emergency.

References

1. Levy D, Larson MG, Vasan RS, et al. The progression from hypertension to congestive heart failure. JAMA. 1996;275:1557.
2. James PA, Oparil S, Carter BL, Cushman WC, Dennison-Himmelfarb C, Handler J, et al. 2014 Evidence-based guideline for the management of high BP in adults: report from the panel members appointed to the Eighth Joint National Committee (JNC 8). JAMA. 2014;311(5):507–20.
3. 2017 ACC/AHA/AAPA/ABC/ACPM/AGS/APhA/ASH/ASPC/NMA/PCNA Guideline for the prevention, detection, evaluation, and management of high blood pressure in adults: a report of the American College of Cardiology/American Heart Association Task Force on Clinical Practice Guidelines.
4. Muntner P, Shimbo D, Carey RM, et al. Measurement of blood pressure in humans: a scientific statement from the American Heart Association. Hypertension. 2019;73:e35.
5. Beevers G, Lip GY, O'Brien E. ABC of hypertension: blood pressure measurement. Part II-conventional sphygmomanometry: technique of auscultatory blood pressure measurement. BMJ. 2001;322:1043.
6. ESH/ESC Task Force for the Management of Arterial Hypertension. 2013 Practice guidelines for the management of arterial hypertension of the European Society of Hypertension (ESH) and the European Society of Cardiology (ESC): ESH/ESC task force for the management of arterial hypertension. J Hypertens. 2013;31(10):1925–38.
7. Shayne PH, Pitts SR. Severely increased BP in the emergency department. Ann Emerg Med. 2003;41(4):513–29.
8. Peixoto AJ. Acute severe hypertension. N Engl J Med. 2019;381:1843.
9. Bianchi S, Bigazzi R, Campese VM. Microalbuminuria in essential hypertension: significance, pathophysiology, and therapeutic implications. Am J Kidney Dis. 1999;34(6):973–95.
10. Staessen JA, Wang J, Bianchi G, Birkenhäger WH. Essential hypertension. Lancet. 2003;361:1629.
11. Wang NY, Young JH, Meoni LA, et al. Blood pressure change and risk of hypertension associated with parental hypertension: the Johns Hopkins Precursors Study. Arch Intern Med. 2008;168:643.
12. Chobanian AV, Bakris GL, Black HR, Cushman WC, Green LA, Izzo JL Jr, National Heart, Lung, and Blood Institute Joint National Committee on Prevention, Detection, Evaluation, and Treatment of High BP; National High BP Education Program Coordinating Committee, et al. The seventh report of the Joint National Committee on prevention, detection, evaluation, and treatment of high BP: the JNC 7 report. JAMA. 2003;289(19):2560–72.
13. Johnson W, Nguyen ML, Patel R. Hypertension crisis in the emergency department. Cardiol Clin. 2012;30(4):533–43.

14. Basile J, Bloch MJ. Overview of hypertension in adults. In: Bakris GL, Kaplan NM, editors. UpTODate. Waltham: UpToDate. http://www.uptodate.com/contents/overview-of-hypertension-in-adults.
15. Eckel RH, Jakicic JM, Ard JD, et al. 2013 AHA/ACC guideline on lifestyle management to reduce cardiovascular risk: a report of the American College of Cardiology/American Heart Association task force on practice guidelines. J Am Coll Cardiol. 2014;63:2960.
16. Williams B, Mancia G, Spiering W, et al. 2018 ESC/ESH guidelines for the management of arterial hypertension. Eur Heart J. 2018;39:3021.
17. Varon J, Elliot WJ. Management of severe asymptomatic hypertension (hypertensive urgencies) in adults. UpToDate; 2021. https://www.uptodate.com/contents/management-of-severe-asymptomat...in-adults/print?search=hypertension&topicRef=3852&source=see_link.
18. Grassi D, O'Flaherty M, Pellizzari M, et al. Hypertensive urgencies in the emergency department: evaluating blood pressure response to rest and to antihypertensive drugs with different profiles. J Clin Hypertens (Greenwich). 2008;10:662.

Gastroesophageal Reflux Disease (GERD) 11

Dipal Shah

11.1 Introduction

Gastroesophageal reflux disease (GERD) is the reflux of gastric content into the esophagus causing discomfort. It is the most commonly diagnosed GI disorder. The exact prevalence of the disease is unclear as the most common symptom, heartburn, is not ubiquitous and therefore will underestimate the prevalence. Additionally, a large subset of patients will have no subjective symptoms at all but will have objective evidence of reflux disease on endoscopy or pH monitoring and thus are underrepresented on survey-based population studies. An Olmsted County survey found 42% of people queried had an episode of heartburn in the preceding year, while 45% noted regurgitation. Of this cohort, approximately 5% visited a physician for the symptoms during this same time period [1].

11.2 History

The diagnosis of GERD can be made by history alone in a patient with the typical symptoms of heartburn and regurgitation, and empiric therapy can be initiated. Given the myriad of over-the-counter (OTC) preparations available, patients have often tired various therapies unsuccessfully prior to seeking medical care. The ineffectiveness of OTC preparations, including proton pump inhibitors (PPIs), does not exclude the diagnosis of GERD, and further investigation is warranted [2].

GERD is typically classified as erosive esophagitis or nonerosive reflux disease based on the appearance of the esophageal mucosa on endoscopy. Erosive esophagitis will show breaks in the distal esophageal mucosa in endoscopy and may or may not have symptoms of GERD. Nonerosive reflux disease (or

D. Shah (✉)
University of Central Florida, Orlando, FL, USA

B. K. Desai et al. (eds.), *Primary Care for Emergency Physicians*,
https://doi.org/10.1007/978-3-031-64676-8_11

endoscopy-negative reflux disease) will have symptoms of GERD with no visible changes to the mucosa on endoscopy.

When chest pain is a presenting symptom, a cardiac etiology should be excluded *prior* to empiric GERD treatment and/or gastrointestinal workup. Thought of a cardiac workup should also be considered for women, who often present with atypical ischemia symptoms, if GERD symptoms are atypical and/or the diagnosis is unclear.

11.3 Risk Factors for GERD

- Obesity, particularly central
- Hiatal hernia
- Pregnancy
- Smoking
- Acid hypersecretion, such as Zollinger-Ellison syndrome
- Lower esophageal dysfunction, such as myotomy
- Dysfunctional esophageal clearance, as with scleroderma
- Delayed gastric emptying as seen in gastroparesis

11.4 Symptoms (Red Flags*)

- Heartburn
- Regurgitation
- Dysphagia*
- Burping
- Dyspepsia (new onset over 60 years*)
- Nausea
- Epigastric pain
- Bloating
- Chest pain
- Bronchospasm
- Odynophagia*
- Sore throat
- Hoarseness
- Globus sensation
- Water brash
- Chronic cough
- Chronic otitis media/sinusitis
- Sleep disturbance
- Weight loss*
- GI bleed*

11.5 Physical Exam

As the esophagus is not directly accessible, the physical evaluation for GERD focuses on evaluating for other possible etiologies particularly for extraesophageal symptoms, when present.

- *Vital signs*
  - Pulse oximetry

GERD is not likely the primary cause of hypoxia but can exacerbate hypoxia in an individual with underlying pulmonary disease.

- *Head, neck, and throat*
  - Laryngeal and pharyngeal inflammation
  - Dental enamel erosion
  - Sinus inflammation
  - Otitis media

The above symptoms are related to chronic recurrent irritation of regurgitated acid resulting in inflammation and hyperplasia.

- *Pulmonary*
  - Wheezing and crackles

Severe GERD can result in primary pulmonary disease but more often triggers an exacerbation of an underlying chronic pulmonary disease.

- *Abdomen*
  - Substernal chest pain or epigastric pain

Possible if GERD is associated with mucosal-based disease like erosive esophagitis or ulceration.

  - Abdominal pain with palpation

Not a common finding and may indicate alternative diagnosis.

  - Bowel sounds

If high-pitched or tympanic sounds present, it may be suggestive of a bowel obstruction, particularly if nausea or vomiting is present.

11.6 Differential Diagnosis

Diagnostic testing is reserved for alarm symptoms, recurrent symptoms, complications or when the diagnosis remains unclear [3].

- Coronary artery disease
- Esophageal disease
  - Esophageal motility disorder
  - Esophageal rings/webs
  - Infectious esophagitis
  - Pill esophagitis
  - Functional esophageal dysfunction
  - Zenker's diverticulum

  - Eosinophilic esophagitis
  - Esophageal cancer
- Gastric disease
  - Gastroparesis
  - Gastritis
  - Peptic ulcer disease
  - Gastric outlet obstruction
- Biliary disease
  - Cholangitis
  - Choledocholithiasis

11.7 Treatment

Treatment of GERD is accomplished via multiple mechanisms: lifestyle modification, creation of a physical barrier, neutralization of acid, blockage of acid production, increase in gastric emptying, and structural enhancement of the gastroesophageal junction. Treatment can be administered on an as-needed basis or chronically depending on their frequency or severity of symptoms. Additional workup is indicated in individuals with alarm symptoms, refractory symptoms, or symptoms that require unusually large doses of medication for control.

- *Lifestyle modification*
  - Avoidance of dietary triggers*
    Caffeine
    Alcohol
    Chocolate
    Peppermint
    Carbonated beverages
    Spicy food
  - Weight loss
  - Avoidance of late night eating, within 3 h of bedtime
  - Elevation of the head of the bed
  - (*Studies are inconsistent regarding benefit; avoidance is recommended based on personal symptom correlation)
- Pharmacologic
  - *Antacids*
    Calcium carbonate
    Aluminum hydroxide
    Over-the-counter formulations used for rapid treatment of acute reflux symptoms by directly neutralizing gastric acid. Onset of action is quick as is the duration of action, 30–60 min. They do not prevent GERD and therefore are only recommended for on-demand use for relief of intermittent GERD symptoms less than once a week.
    Pitfalls

1. Diarrhea
2. Renal impairment
3. Electrolyte abnormalities

– *Mucosal-based agent*

Aluminum sucrose sulfate

Directly coats the esophageal mucosa creating a physical barrier to gastric content promoting healing. This agent is useful in the treatment of mild reflux disease as well as for use in pregnancy, Category B.

Pitfalls

1. Caution in renal insufficiency
2. Aluminum toxicity
3. Hypophosphatemia

Bismuth subsalicylate

Over-the-counter preparation used for treatment of mild to moderate reflux symptoms. It has antisecretory properties and provides a direct mucosa barrier. It is useful for its rapid onset but has a short duration of action. Its antimicrobial effects are adjunctive in the treatment of *H. pylori*.

Pitfalls

1. Blackened stool, which can be confused with melena
2. Bismuth toxicity

– *Histamine-2 receptor antagonists*

Famotidine
Cimetidine
Ranitidine
Nizatidine

Over-the-counter preparations used for treatment of mild to moderate reflux, which work by blocking the histamine-2 receptor on parietal cells, thereby decreasing acid secretion. Useful for on-demand treatment of reflux symptoms and can be taken once or twice daily for long-term therapy. Nocturnal dosing can be considered in patients with persistent symptoms, nighttime symptoms, despite daily PPI usage. Ranitidine and cimetidine felt to be safe for use in pregnancy, Category B [4]. They are typically ineffective for severe erosive esophagitis.

Pitfalls

1. Tachyphylaxis limits effectiveness to 6–8 weeks of usage.
2. Require dose reduction for renal insufficiency.
3. Myelosuppression.
4. Gynecomastia.
5. Impotence.
6. Hepatitis.
7. Multiple drug–drug interactions, primarily with cimetidine.

– *Proton pump inhibitors*

Omeprazole*
Omeprazole/sodium bicarbonate*

Rabeprazole
Esomeprazole
Pantoprazole
Lansoprazole*
Dexlansoprazole

The antacid effect of this group is obtained by direct irreversible inhibition of the hydrogen-potassium ATPase pump located on parietal cell. As a group, they are the most effective pharmacologic antacid therapy available. There are seven formulations that are effectively equivalent in efficacy on a milligram per milligram basis. Three formulations are available over the counter,* while the others require a prescription. Once-daily AM dosing is recommended with an increase in frequency, change in administration time, or change in formulation based on an individual's response. They are administered 30–60 min prior to a meal and may take up to 5 days before maximal effect is demonstrated. Chronic therapy is indicated in patients with recurrent symptoms with discontinuation and/or complications related to reflux like erosive esophagitis, strictures, or Barrett's esophagus. The lowest effective dose should be used for long-term maintenance [2].

Pitfalls

1. Short-term use may increase the risk of community- and hospital-acquired pneumonia.
2. There may be increase in the risk of *Clostridium difficile* infection in at-risk patients.
3. Discontinuation in patients with osteoporosis *not* indicated, although therapy may increase the risk of hip fracture or additional bone loss in the setting of other risk factors for hip fracture and change in therapy should be considered.
4. No alteration of therapy indicated for concomitant clopidogrel usage.
5. Potential calcium, iron, and vitamin B12 malabsorption.

11.8 Treatment Failures

Medically refractory symptoms require additional workup and specialty evaluation. Risk factors that predict treatment failure include a family history of GERD, dose escalation of antacid therapy, inability to discontinue antacid therapy, esophagitis on endoscopy, and failure of esophagitis to heal despite adequate therapy [5].

- Diagnostic evaluation
  - *Esophagram*

    Allows evaluation for mass, strictures, and stenosis; often deferred in place of endoscopy which allows for treatment and tissue sampling

    Recommended prior to endoluminal or surgical therapy to define anatomy: hernias, diverticula, etc.
  - *Endoscopy*

    - Allows for assessment severity of disease
        - Esophagitis
        - Strictures/stenosis
        - Barrett's esophagus
    - Evaluation for alternate diagnoses
        - Eosinophilic esophagitis
        - Malignancy
        - Gastric outlet obstruction
  - *Gastric emptying study*
    - Evaluation for delayed gastric emptying
  - *Ambulatory reflux monitoring*
    - Documents acid exposure and regurgitation events
        - Documents the presence of disease in patients without esophagitis
    - Correlates symptoms with reflux episodes
    - Documents in/effectiveness of medication
  - *Esophageal manometry*
    - Not required for diagnosis or evaluation of refractory symptoms but necessary prior to consideration of endoluminal or surgical treatment for reflux
    - Documents adequate esophageal motility
    - Detects early achalasia, disorder often confused with GERD
- Nonpharmacologic intervention
  - *Endoluminal therapy*
  - Two presently FDA-approved therapies: Stretta and transoral incisionless fundoplication (TIF). Short-term results are promising, but long-term efficacy remains to be seen [2].
    - Stretta
        - Applies radiofrequency energy to the esophagus causing inflammation and fibrosis resulting in decreased tissue compliance and lower esophageal sphincter relaxation
    - TIF
        - Endoscopically creates a reflux barrier similar to traditional surgical fundoplications
  - *Surgery*
  - Shown to be equally effective as medical management in the appropriately chosen patient population for the control of GERD symptoms [6]. However, long-term efficacy has not been established.
    - Fundoplication
        - Recreates and/or augments the physical barrier at the lower esophagus
        - Exact type of surgery dependent upon surgeon expertise and patient characteristics

References

1. Richter JE. In: Yamada T, editor. Textbook of gastroenterology. Hoboken: Blackwell's Publishing; 2009.
2. Katz PO, Gerson LB, Vela MF. Guidelines for the diagnosis and management of gastroesophageal reflux disease. Am J Gastroenterol. 2013;108:308–26.
3. Tytgat GN. Review article: Treatment of mild and severe cases of GERD. Aliment Pharmacol Ther. 2002;16(Suppl. 4):73–8.
4. McGuigan JE, Belafsky PC, Fromer L, Mccarthy D, Nostrant T, Postma GN, et al. Review article: Diagnosis and management of night-time reflux. Aliment Pharmacol Ther. 2004;20(Suppl. 9):57–72.
5. Worrell SG, Greene CL, DeMeester TR. The state of surgical treatment of gastroesophageal reflux disease after five decades. J Am Coll Surg. 2014;219(4):819–30.
6. SAGES Guidelines Committee. Guidelines for surgical treatment of gastroesophageal reflux disease (GERD). Society of America Gastrointestinal and Endoscopic Surgeons; 2010. www.sages.org.

Dyspnea

12

Alpa Desai

12.1 Introduction

Dyspnea is defined by an official statement of the American Thoracic Society as "a subjective experience of breathing discomfort that consists of qualitatively distinct sensations that vary in intensity" [1]. A wide variety of patient complaints can therefore fall under the umbrella of dyspnea, including shortness of death, chest tightness, and a sense of impending doom [2]. The associated differential diagnosis ranges from minor self-limited etiologies to the immediately life-threatening. Unfortunately, there is often poor correlation with the severity of self-reported dyspnea and the seriousness of the underlying etiology [3].

12.2 Differential Diagnosis

- Cardiopulmonary
  - Acute coronary syndrome (ACS)
  - Airway obstruction
    - Airway infections (epiglottitis, retropharyngeal abscess)
    - Anaphylaxis
    - Angioedema
    - Foreign body
    - Hemorrhage
  - Arrhythmia
  - Asthma
  - Chronic obstructive pulmonary disease (COPD)
  - Malignancy

A. Desai (✉)
Department of Community Health and Family Medicine, University of Florida College of Medicine, Gainesville, FL, USA

B. K. Desai et al. (eds.), *Primary Care for Emergency Physicians*,
https://doi.org/10.1007/978-3-031-64676-8_12

  - Pericardial disease (effusion, pericarditis, tamponade)
  - Pleural effusion
  - Pneumonia
  - Pulmonary embolus (PE)
  - Pulmonary edema/congestive heart failure (CHF)
  - Spontaneous pneumothorax
  - Valvular dysfunction
- Abdominal
  - Ascites
  - Obesity
  - Pregnancy
  - Referred pain
- Hematologic/metabolic
  - Acute chest syndrome
  - Anemia
  - Carbon monoxide poisoning
  - Diabetic ketoacidosis
  - Fever
  - Organophosphate poisoning
  - Renal failure
  - Salicylate overdose
  - Sepsis
  - Thyrotoxicosis
- Neuromuscular
  - Botulism
  - Cerebrovascular accident
  - Guillain-Barre syndrome
  - Myasthenia gravis
- Psychiatric
  - Hyperventilation
  - Somatization
- Traumatic
  - Cardiac tamponade
  - Flail chest
  - Hemothorax
  - Pneumothorax
  - Pulmonary contusion
  - Rib fractures

12.3 History

When obtaining the history in a patient presenting with dyspnea, the clinician should focus not only on obvious respiratory symptoms but also on symptoms referable to interrelated organ systems, particularly the cardiovascular and renal systems.

Neurologic, gastrointestinal, and psychiatric conditions can also lead to chief complaint of dyspnea. Any history of recent traumatic injury should also be elicited. With regard to the past medical history, focus on preexisting cardiopulmonary conditions as well as smoking history, occupational exposure history, and risk factors for ACS and PE (discussed below).

- Temporal course of symptoms
  - Abrupt worsening (*red flag): PE, flash pulmonary edema, and spontaneous pneumothorax
  - Gradual onset: pneumonia, CHF exacerbation, and anemia
- Triggers of dyspnea
  - Allergens
  - Environmental pollutants: asthma and COPD exacerbation
  - Exertion: ACS and CHF
  - Paroxysmal nocturnal dyspnea and orthopnea: CHF
- Wheezing
- Stridor
- Cough
- Quality
  - "Barking": croup
  - Sputum: COPD ± acute exacerbation and pneumonia
  - Hemoptysis (*red flag): tuberculosis, malignancy, or PE
- Associated symptoms
  - Abdominal pain
  - Anxiety/depression
  - Ascending muscle weakness: Guillain-Barre
  - Chest pain (*red flag)
  - Edema of the face, abdomen, or legs: renal failure, liver failure and CHF
  - Unilateral leg swelling (*red flag): venous thromboembolism
  - Fever
  - Leg pain (*red flag): venous thromboembolism
  - Weight gain: renal failure and CHF
  - Weight loss: malignancy and thyrotoxicosis

12.4 Physical

In any patient with a complaint of dyspnea, it is necessary to immediately evaluate for signs of impending respiratory failure.

*Red flags for impending respiratory failure:

- Accessory muscle use
- Paradoxical respiration
- Bilateral absent breath sounds
- Stridor

- Altered mental status
- Tripoding
- Inability to handle secretions

Once the need for emergent airway or respiratory interventions has been excluded, the exam can turn to a more systematic approach to gather further clues to the etiology of dyspnea.

- Oropharyngeal exam
  - Oropharyngeal edema/obstruction (*red flag)
  - Respiratory exam
- Barrel chest: COPD
- Pursed lip breathing
- Auscultation:
  - Absent breath sounds (*red flag)
  - Decreased breath sounds:
    - Bilateral (*red flag): severe asthma or COPD exacerbation and bilateral pleural effusions
    - Unilateral: pneumothorax and unilateral effusion
    - Wheezes: asthma, CHF, and COPD
    - Crackles/rales: PNA and CHF
  - Stridor (*red flag): croup, retropharyngeal abscess, and anaphylaxis
- Cardiovascular exam
  - Jugular venous distention (*red flag): CHF, tension pneumothorax, pericardial tamponade
  - Muffled heart sounds (*red flag): pericardial effusion with or without tamponade
  - S3 or S4: heart failure
- Abdominal exam: evaluate for intra-abdominal pathology which may irritate the diaphragm or cause apparent respiratory difficulty
  - Distention
  - Tenderness
- Dermatologic exam
  - Clubbing
  - Cyanosis
  - Dependent edema: CHF and renal failure

12.5 Specific Relevant Etiologies

12.5.1 Asthma

The prevalence of asthma among Americans is approximately 8%, with slightly higher rates among children. In 2008, approximately half of patients with asthma reported having at least one attack [4], making asthma exacerbations one of the most frequent emergency department diagnoses. While the details of the pathophysiology are complex, the condition is ultimately the result of an abnormal inflammatory response resulting in airway obstruction due to smooth muscle constriction, airway edema, and accumulation of secretions. Exacerbations are typically associated with dyspnea, chest tightness, wheezing, and/or cough. In addition to standard historical data mentioned above, clinicians should inquire regarding potential triggers of symptoms, as well as any history of intensive care unit admissions, history of intubation, and personal best measures on peak expiratory flow (PEF) testing.

Labs and imaging are of limited value in patients with a known history of asthma presenting with an uncomplicated exacerbation. The severity of illness and response to treatment is best assessed by clinical judgment and PEF testing, which is widely available in EDs and primary care offices, in contrast to spirometry. Values obtained by individuals can be compared to age-, sex-, and height-matched predicted values to monitor the severity of an exacerbation as well as the response to treatment. Severe exacerbations are typically defined by a PEF reading <40% of personal best or predicted, with mild exacerbations by a reading ≥70% of these values. Moderate-severity exacerbations comprise the remainder.

Inhaled β-agonists are a cornerstone of asthma therapy. These agents relax bronchial smooth muscle, resulting in bronchodilation. Albuterol, a short-acting, rapid-onset, β2-selective agent, is typically the drug of choice for acute exacerbations. Albuterol can be administered via metered dose inhaler (with or without a spacer device) or via nebulization. In the hospital setting, treatments are often delivered via nebulizer and can be given continuously or on a periodic basis. In the home setting, for children older than 1 year of age, there is no apparent benefit to nebulized therapy versus a metered dose inhaler with spacer. Levalbuterol does not appear to convey any benefit with respect to safety or efficacy compared with albuterol but does cost significantly more. Combination of inhaled ipratropium with albuterol may reduce the need for hospitalization in patients with severe exacerbations. Systemic β-agonists do not appear beneficial compared with inhaled agents [5].

Early administration of systemic corticosteroids (40–60 mg prednisone PO for adults or 1–2 mg/kg prednisolone PO for children, or 1 mg/kg methylprednisolone IV) reduces the rate of hospitalization. Patients are typically prescribed a non-tapering course of a total of 3–10 days of 40–60 mg prednisone daily (1–2 mg/kg prednisolone in children) once discharged from the ED or inpatient hospitalization. Prednisolone is preferred in children due to its palatability relative to prednisone.

Magnesium administration (25–75 mg/kg in children, up to 2 mg IV in adults) may be considered in severe exacerbations. Methylxanthines, such as theophylline, have a narrow therapeutic index and are generally avoided. Heliox has not proven to be effective in improving relevant clinical endpoints.

Long-acting β-agonists, such as salmeterol and formoterol, are indicated for maintenance therapy in patients with persistent asthma (generally defined as symptoms typically present for >2 days/week). These agents should not be used as an alternative to short-acting β-agonists in patients with acute exacerbations. Commercially available preparations of long-acting agents often also contain an inhaled corticosteroid (examples include budesonide/formoterol, mometasone/formoterol, and salmeterol/fluticasone).

Leukotriene-modifying agents, such as montelukast, zafirlukast, and zileuton, are useful as a potential alternative to inhaled corticosteroids in patients with persistent asthma. These agents are not indicated for use in acute exacerbations.

Patients with continued symptoms and/or a PEF <40% following initial ED treatment should be admitted to the hospital for continued care. Patients with a sustained good response to therapy (PEF ≥ 70% and improved symptoms) can generally be discharged. In the remainder of patients, a case-by case decision should be made, with careful consideration of the severity of patient's prior exacerbations, comorbidities, access to primary care, and social supports. In discharged patients, a continued course of systemic steroids is indicated as noted above. Ensure that adequate supplies of short-acting β-agonist are available, give complete return precautions, and ensure prompt follow-up with the patient's PCP. In patients with a history of persistent asthma, consider addition of an inhaled steroid if not already utilized [3, 5].

12.5.2 COPD Exacerbations

The prevalence of COPD among American adults is approximately 6%, with approximately 19% of those affected reporting at least one ED visit or hospitalization in the previous year [6]. COPD is classically divided into chronic bronchitis and emphysema, although significant overlap exists between these forms (chronic obstructive asthma and bronchiectasis are also considered forms of COPD). Chronic bronchitis is defined clinically as the presence of a productive cough for at least 3 months in 2 consecutive years without an alternative explanation. Emphysema is defined by the destruction of distal airways, including bronchioles and alveoli, without evidence of fibrosis. In each form, there exists persistent airflow limitation and an abnormal inflammatory response. Smoking is by far the leading risk factor, although α-1 antitrypsin deficiency and exposure to occupational and environmental pollutants are also associated. At the time of diagnosis, patients typically report chronic and progressive dyspnea and cough with or without sputum production. The formal diagnosis of COPD is made by spirometry based on a post-bronchodilator forced expiratory volume in 1 s/forced vital capacity (FEV_1/FVC) of <0.70. Further stratification of the severity can be made by the GOLD criteria (Table 12.1) [7].

COPD exacerbations are characterized by an acute change in sputum character or an increase in dyspnea, cough, or sputum volume. A host of causes exists, with viral and bacterial infections by far the most common triggers. Environmental

Table 12.1 Severity of airflow limitation according to the GOLD criteria

Severity	FEV_1 (% predicted)
Mild	≥80%
Moderate	50–79%
Severe	30–49%
Very severe	<30%

respiratory irritants, PE, pneumothorax, CHF, β-blocker use, and cold weather have also been implicated. Frequently, no cause is identified.

12.6 Chronic Management

The acute management of COPD exacerbations is quite analogous to that of asthma exacerbations. A key distinguishing factor is the relative lack of acute reversibility of airflow obstruction, limiting the utility of PEF measurement and reassessments in these patients.

Supplemental oxygen should be administered to maintain saturations of at least 90%. Additional doses of short-acting β-agonist, combined with an inhaled anticholinergic agent (albuterol/ipratropium) beyond the patient's baseline regimen, are generally indicated. Oral steroids such as prednisone (or methylprednisolone IV in patients unable to tolerate PO) are also of benefit. A key distinction from acute asthma management is the role of antibiotics. As bacterial infection (particularly *Streptococcus pneumoniae*, *Haemophilus influenzae*, and *Moraxella catarrhalis*) is commonly associated with the development of COPD exacerbations, patients with increased sputum production and/or moderate to severe exacerbations should typically be prescribed antibiotics. There is no clear data to support the use of any particular agent. Antimicrobial choice should therefore be guided by local resistance patterns to the above pathogens. Commonly utilized antibiotics include amoxicillin ± clavulanate, doxycycline, azithromycin, and respiratory fluoroquinolones. The optimal duration of antimicrobial treatment is also unclear [8]. Intravenous magnesium can also be considered in severe exacerbations, although evidence supporting its use is lacking. Long-acting inhaled anticholinergics (tiotropium and aclidinium) and inhaled corticosteroids (beclomethasone, budesonide, ciclesonide, fluticasone, and mometasone, often combined with long-acting β-agonists as described in the asthma section), while beneficial in chronic management of COPD, are not of benefit in the setting of an acute exacerbation [9].

Patients with marked worsening from baseline (such as new or increasing oxygen requirements), those who fail to improve (or worsen) despite the above interventions, and those with significant comorbidities or inadequate social support (including poor access to medications or primary care follow-up) should be admitted. If the decision is made to discharge a patient with a COPD exacerbation, ensure adequate supplies of albuterol with or without ipratropium are available to the patient, as well as sufficient amounts of supplemental home oxygen and any additional medications prescribed for COPD by their primary care physician. A several-day course of oral steroids is generally indicated, analogous to asthma management. If indicated, prescribe an appropriate antibiotic regimen. Finally, counsel patients who continue to smoke regarding the role of smoking cessation in the chronic management of COPD, as it is the only intervention shown to favorably alter the course of the disease [9].

12.6.1 Hyperventilation

Hyperventilation refers to minute ventilation in excess of metabolic needs. Anxiety disorders, including panic disorder, are commonly associated. The diagnosis should be one of exclusion, after careful consideration of the numerous potentially life-threatening etiologies of dyspnea noted above. Patients may report associated feelings of impending doom, palpitations, paresthesias, presyncope, chest pain, diaphoresis, and carpopedal spasm. An inciting distressing event may also be reported. Once emergent diagnoses have been excluded, a small dose of a benzodiazepine, such as lorazepam, may be considered for resolution of an acute episode. Rebreathing of CO_2 (such as via a paper bag) was once widely advocated as a remedy for acute hyperventilation. However, due to concerns regarding potential hypoxemia, this treatment modality should be avoided [10]. If episodes are recurrent, treatment of any underlying anxiety disorder should be the focus of therapy as outlined in the chapter on anxiety.

12.6.2 Croup

Inflammation of the larynx and subglottic airway due to viral or bacterial illness resulting in stridor and cough is termed croup. Parainfluenza viruses are the most common culprit, although respiratory syncytial virus and influenza viruses are also implicated. Children between the ages of 6 months and 3 years are most commonly affected, with peak incidence in late fall, early winter, and spring. The course of illness typically begins with several days of URI symptoms such as congestion, rhinorrhea, and fever, followed by the onset of the typical barking cough, stridor, and hoarseness, which usually abates within 48 h. Young children are much more severely affected due to narrow caliber of the airway in this age group, whereas adults typically only experience the hoarseness attributed to "laryngitis." Treatment for all pediatric patients presenting with croup includes immediate assessment of the ability to protect their airway, followed by administration of oral steroids. Dexamethasone (0.6 mg/kg, max 10 mg) is the preferred agent given its prolonged half-life. Oral administration is as effective as parenteral and has the advantage of being less alarming to a child than an injection, which could induce further respiratory difficulty. In patients with moderate (stridor at rest, frequent barking cough, chest wall retractions) to severe croup (respiratory distress, marked retraction, inspiratory and expiratory stridor), nebulized epinephrine should be administered. If clinical response is noted, patients should be observed for approximately 4 h as the potential for rebound symptoms exists. Patients with persistent increased work of breathing or stridor at rest, as well as those requiring more than two doses of epinephrine, should be admitted.

12.6.3 Pulmonary Embolism

Pulmonary embolism (PE) is a feared cause of dyspnea with a significant burden of mortality. It has been estimated that up to 100,000 Americans die each year from PE [11], and fear of missing the diagnosis fuels a significant number of evaluations for the condition. The presentation varies from sudden cardiac death to incidentally diagnosed PE in virtually asymptomatic patients. The most common symptoms include dyspnea, pleuritic chest pain, leg pain/swelling, and cough (with or without hemoptysis). The onset of symptoms is often rapid, although significant variation exists. Tachycardia, hypoxemia, tachypnea, and leg tenderness and swelling may be noted on physical exam. Risk factors for PE include the components of Virchow's triad: venous stasis (prolonged immobilization), thrombophilia (e.g., malignancy, inherited thrombophilias, use of exogenous estrogens), and vascular endothelial injury.

CT pulmonary angiography (CTPA) is the most commonly used imaging study to confirm the diagnosis of PE, although ventilation/perfusion scanning is utilized in some pregnant patients, as well as in patients with contrast allergies and renal insufficiency. The sensitivity and specificity of CTPA are excellent. However, CTPA does expose patients to a significant amount of radiation and nephrotoxic contrast dye. Therefore, appropriate selection of patients for this testing is key. The pulmonary embolism rule-out criteria (PERC rule) identify patients for whom no further testing is indicated. To fulfill the rule, the clinician must estimate a low pretest probability of PE (<15%), and the patient must fulfill all of the criteria listed below [12]:

- Age <50
- Pulse rate <100
- Room air oxygen saturation ≥95%
- Absence of hemoptysis
- No use of exogenous estrogens
- No history of venous thromboembolism
- No surgery or trauma in the past 4 weeks
- Absence of unilateral leg swelling

In patients for whom PE cannot be excluded by the PERC rule, an estimation of pretest probability should be made, either by clinician gestalt or by a structured decision rule such as the Wells score [13]. Patients with a high pretest probability (e.g., Wells score >4 [14]) should proceed directly to a definitive imaging study, while those with a low pretest probability are appropriate for D-dimer testing as a first step. Those patients with a D-dimer below the test threshold are considered to have PE effectively excluded, while others should proceed to definitive imaging.

Presently, treatment of confirmed PE generally includes hospitalization and initiation of anticoagulation with heparin, low-molecular weight heparin, or fondaparinux. Patients are then typically transitioned to oral anticoagulants such as warfarin, rivaroxaban, apixaban, or edoxaban. Hypotensive patients without contraindications should be strongly considered for thrombolysis. Thrombolysis in patients with evidence of right ventricular strain (hypokinesis or dilatation, troponinemia, or brain natriuretic peptide elevation) is controversial.

12.6.4 Pneumonia

Approximately four million cases of community-acquired pneumonia (CAP) are diagnosed per year [15]. Many additional patients are diagnosed with healthcare-associated pneumonia (HCAP) or hospital-acquired pneumonia. The first two entities are of particular relevance to emergency and outpatient-based primary care physicians. Cough is present in nearly all patients, with dyspnea, sputum production, and chest pain also frequently reported. Elderly patients often report fewer or atypical symptoms, so a lower threshold to evaluate for pneumonia is warranted in this population. On physical exam, fever, tachycardia, tachypnea, hypoxemia, rales, wheezes, and/or diminished lung sounds may be appreciated. A chest X-ray should be obtained in patients with clinical evidence of pneumonia, and, strictly speaking, a demonstrable infiltrate must be present to make the diagnosis [16].

HCAP is defined as a pneumonia diagnosis in a patient who has been hospitalized for 2 or more days within the past 90 days, is a resident of a nursing home or long-term care facility, has received care at a hemodialysis clinic in the past 30 days, or has received wound care, IV chemotherapy, or other IV infusions in the past 30 days [17]. Outpatients with none of these features are classified as having CAP. The distinction is important, as the potential for multiple drug-resistant bacterial infection is quite significant in patients with HCAP.

Common identified etiologies of CAP include *Mycoplasma pneumoniae*, *Chlamydophila pneumoniae*, *S. pneumoniae*, *H. influenzae*, and respiratory viruses, such as influenza, adenovirus, and respiratory syncytial virus. Atypical pathogens such as *Mycoplasma* and *Chlamydophila* are commonly associated with milder disease ("walking pneumonia") outbreaks in crowded facilities such as college dormitories. Chest X-ray in these patients often reveals an interstitial pattern. Tuberculosis is commonly associated with upper lobe involvement on chest X-ray, cavitating lesions, and mediastinal lymphadenopathy. *Legionella* should be considered in patients with high fever, gastrointestinal symptoms, relative bradycardia, smoking history, and underlying lung disease. Urine antigen testing can be used to identify infected patients.

Several methods exist to risk-stratify disposition decisions for adult patients with community-acquired pneumonia. The Pneumonia Severity Index, which has been extensively studied and externally validated, stratifies patients into one of five risk classifications with 30-day mortality risks ranging between 0.1 and 27.0% [18]. A number of elements of historical and laboratory data are required, and the calculation can be somewhat cumbersome, so the use of an online calculator is typically employed to aid in appropriate classification. A simpler alternative method is the CURB-65 rule, which stratifies patients on the basis of confusion, urea (BUN >20 mg/dL), respiratory rate ≥30/min, BP (systolic < 90 or diastolic ≤60 mmHg), and age ≥65 years. Reported 30-day mortality rates range from 0.7 to 57% in patients with 0 to 5 factors, respectively [19]. As is the case with any decision rule, clinical judgment must always supersede. Hypoxic patients, particularly those with an oxygen saturation < 92%, should be strongly considered for admission regardless of results of formal risk stratification results [20]. In the pediatric population, infants under the age of 3–6 months and children with significant cardiopulmonary comorbidities, respiratory distress, hypoxemia, toxic appearance, and poor feeding should generally be hospitalized.

If treating as an outpatient, typical regimens for CAP adults include a macrolide such as azithromycin or a respiratory fluoroquinolone such as levofloxacin. If significant local resistance of *S. pneumoniae* to macrolides exists, macrolide monotherapy should not be used. Atypical pathogens are uncommon in children beyond infancy and less than 5 years old; therefore, high-dose amoxicillin is typical first-line coverage. The increasing prevalence of atypical infections in older children results in macrolides being appropriate empiric therapy for this population. Patients hospitalized for CAP are typically started on either a respiratory fluoroquinolone or the combination of a parenteral third-generation cephalosporin (such as ceftriaxone) as well as a macrolide. Patients requiring ICU-level care are generally empirically started on more aggressive antibiotic regimens. Regardless of age group or disposition decision, it is always wise to consider the possibility of influenza pneumonia and possible treatment with oseltamivir. If suspicion for tuberculosis exists, place the patient in respiratory isolation, admit the patient, and obtain acid-fast stains of the sputum. Patients with healthcare-associated pneumonia should be admitted and placed on broad-spectrum antibiotics as the potential for resistant bacterial infection is quite significant. Treatment should include coverage for *Pseudomonas aeruginosa* as well as MRSA.

Discharged patients should have close follow-up arranged, and any worsening or failure to improve within 48–72 h should prompt consideration of hospital admission and broadening of antibiotic coverage.

References

1. Parshall MB, Schwartzstein RM, Adams L, Banzett RB, Manning HL, et al. An official American Thoracic Society statement: update on the mechanisms, assessment, and management of dyspnea. Am J Respir Crit Care Med. 2012;185:435–52.
2. Banzett RB, Schwartzstein RM. Dyspnea: don't just look, ask! Am J Respir Crit Care Med. 2015;192:1404–6.
3. Marx JA, Hockberger RS, Walls RM. Rosen's emergency medicine—concepts and clinical practice. 8th ed. Philadelphia: Elsevier Saunders; 2013.
4. Centers for Disease Control and Prevention. Vital signs: asthma prevalence, disease characteristics, and self-management education: United States, 2001–2009. MMWR Morb Mortal Wkly Rep. 2011;60:547–52.
5. Pollart SM, Compton RM, Elward KS. Management of acute asthma exacerbations. Am Fam Physician. 2011;84:40–7.
6. Centers for Disease Control and Prevention. Chronic obstructive pulmonary disease among adults—United States, 2011. MMWR Morb Mortal Wkly Rep. 2012;61:938–43.

7. Global strategy for the diagnosis, management and prevention of COPD. Global Initiative for Chronic Obstructive Lung Disease (GOLD); 2016. http://www.goldcopd.org/guidelines-global-strategy-for-diagnosis-management.html.
8. Vollenweider DJ, Jarrett H, Steurer-Stey CA, Garcia-Aymerich J, Puhan MA. Antibiotics for exacerbations of chronic obstructive pulmonary disease. Cochrane Database Syst Rev. 2012;12:CD010257.
9. Evensen AE. Management of COPD exacerbations. Am Fam Physician. 2010;81:607–13.
10. Callaham M. Hypoxic hazards of traditional paper bag rebreathing in hyperventilating patients. Ann Emerg Med. 1989;18:622–8.
11. Horlander KT, Mannino DM, Leeper KV. Pulmonary embolism mortality in the United States, 1979-1998: an analysis using multiple-cause mortality data. Arch Intern Med. 2003;163:1711–7.
12. Kline JA, Courtney DM, Kabrhel C, Moore CL, Smithline HA, et al. Prospective multicenter evaluation of the pulmonary embolism rule-out criteria. J Thromb Haemost. 2008;6:772–80.
13. Wells PS, Anderson DR, Rodger M, Ginsberg JS, Kearon C, et al. Derivation of a simple clinical model to categorize patients probability of pulmonary embolism: increasing the models utility with the SimpliRED D-dimer. Thromb Haemost. 2000;83:416–20.
14. van Belle A, Büller HR, Huisman MV, Huisman PM, Kaasjager K, et al.; Christopher Study Investigators. Effectiveness of managing suspected pulmonary embolism using an algorithm combining clinical probability, D-dimer testing, and computed tomography. JAMA. 2006;295:172–179.
15. Halm EA, Teirstein AS. Management of community-acquired pneumonia. N Engl J Med. 2002;347:2039–45.
16. Mandell LA, Wunderink RG, Anzueto A, Bartlett JG, Campbell GD, Dean NC, Dowell SF, File TM Jr, Musher DM, Niederman MS, Torres A, Whitney CG, Infectious Diseases Society of America; American Thoracic Society. Infectious Diseases Society of America/American Thoracic Society consensus guidelines on the management of community-acquired pneumonia in adults. Clin Infect Dis. 2007;44:S27–72.
17. American Thoracic Society, Infectious Diseases Society of America. Guidelines for the management of adults with hospital-acquired, ventilator-associated, and healthcare-associated pneumonia. Am J Respir Crit Care Med. 2005;171(4):388–416.
18. Fine MJ, Auble TE, Yealy DM, Hanusa BH, Weissfeld LA, Singer DE, Coley CM, Marrie TJ, Kapoor WN. A prediction rule to identify low-risk patients with community-acquired pneumonia. N Engl J Med. 1997;336:243–50.
19. Lim WS, van der Eerden MM, Laing R, Boersma WG, Karalus N, Town GI, Lewis SA, Macfarlane JT. Defining community acquired pneumonia severity on presentation to hospital: an international derivation and validation study. Thorax. 2003;58:377–82.
20. Majumdar SR, Eurich DT, Gamble JM, Senthilselvan A, Marrie TJ. Oxygen saturations less than 92% are associated with major adverse events in outpatients with pneumonia: a population-based cohort study. Clin Infect Dis. 2011;52:325–31.

Hemoptysis

13

Emily Macauley and James Link Wilson

13.1 Introduction

Hemoptysis can be defined as the expectoration of blood that originates from the lower respiratory tract below the glottis (trachea, bronchi, and bronchioles) [1]. The majority of cases of hemoptysis seen in the emergency department involve trace losses of blood and are not life-threatening. Less than 5% of patients will present with massive hemoptysis which is generally defined as over 200 mL of blood loss over a 24-h period or more than 100 mL within an hour [2]. The exact amount of blood is difficult to quantify in the clinical setting; therefore, it is more common to use the volume as a factor in decision-making. Additional considerations should be made for the briskness of bleeding, ability of a patient to maintain a patent airway and expectorate blood, and the patient's underlying physiologic reserve [3]. Mortality associated with hemoptysis is typically not hemorrhagic shock but instead asphyxiation from hemorrhage flooding the airways or inability to oxygenate [3]. Massive hemoptysis can cause hemodynamic changes resulting in inadequate gas exchange and reaches a mortality rate of 75% [4]. Therefore, massive hemoptysis requires prompt intervention to ensure airway protection and adequate ventilation.

Care must also be given to determining other potential sources of bleeding. Bleeding from the nasopharynx, oropharynx, or gastrointestinal system can often mimic true hemoptysis as blood can sometimes contaminate the tracheobronchial tree.

Hemoptysis is rare in the pediatric population, but causes can include lower respiratory tract infections, irritation from aspiration of foreign bodies, congenital heart disease, and bronchiectasis (typically associated with cystic fibrosis) [5].

E. Macauley (✉) · J. L. Wilson
University of Central Florida, Orlando, FL, USA

B. K. Desai et al. (eds.), *Primary Care for Emergency Physicians*,
https://doi.org/10.1007/978-3-031-64676-8_13

13.2 Pathophysiology

The blood supply to the lungs is made up primarily by two arterial vascular systems:

- The bronchial arteries carry oxygenated blood to the lung parenchyma. These arteries branch from the aorta and are at systemic pressure.
- The pulmonary arteries are responsible for bringing deoxygenated blood to the lung for gas exchange and are under much lower pressures [6].

Approximately 90% of massive hemoptysis arises from the bronchial arteries, while 5% originates from the pulmonary arteries [7]. Episodes of low-volume hemoptysis tend to arise from capillaries that are disrupted due to trauma, inflammation, infection, or even infarction [6].

13.3 Risk Factors

Risk factors for significant hemoptysis are similar to risk factors for lung cancer:

- Smoking
- Age greater than 40
- Anticoagulant use
- Asbestos exposure
- Travel
  - Increased risk of developing pulmonary embolism
  - Exposure to tuberculosis

13.4 Differential Diagnosis

- Pseudohemoptysis
  - Nasopharyngeal bleeding
  - Oropharyngeal bleeding
  - Gastrointestinal bleeding
- Tracheobronchial sources
  - Bronchitis—accounts for up to half of cases of hemoptysis
    - Acute
    - Chronic
  - Bronchiectasis
  - Cystic fibrosis
  - Neoplasm
    - Small cell carcinoma
    - Squamous cell carcinoma
    - Bronchial adenoma
    - Metastatic disease

        - Carcinoid tumor
        - Kaposi's sarcoma
    - Traumatic injury to the airway
    - Foreign body
    - Broncholithiasis
- Parenchymal sources
    - Pneumonia
        - *Staphylococcus*
        - *Legionella*
        - Pneumococcus
        - *Klebsiella*
    - Tuberculosis—accounts for a small minority in the United States but remains the most common cause in third world countries [6]
    - Viral
        - Varicella
        - Influenza
    - Fungal
        - *Aspergillus*
        - *Coccidioides*
        - *Histoplasma*
        - *Blastomyces*
    - Pneumonitis
        - Inhalational
        - Chemical
    - Lung abscess
    - Lung contusion
    - Goodpasture syndrome
    - Wegener's granulomatosis
- Vascular sources
    - Congestive heart failure
    - Arteriovenous malformation
    - Aortopulmonary fistula
    - Aortic aneurysm
    - Pulmonary embolism
    - Pulmonary hypertension
    - Endocarditis
    - Mitral stenosis
- Coagulation sources
    - Von Willebrand disease
    - Thrombocytopenia
    - Hemophilia
    - Antiplatelet or anticoagulant use
    - Disseminated intravascular coagulation
- Other sources
    - Iatrogenic

    - Tracheostomy/intubation complications
    - Post-bronchoscopy
    - Post-biopsy
    - Pulmonary artery catheter
  - Autoimmune
    - Behcet's disease
    - SLE
    - Polyarteritis nodosa
  - Ectopic endometrial tissue
  - Trauma
  - Illegal drugs
    - Marijuana
    - Cocaine
  - Idiopathic

Conditions which are more likely to cause massive hemoptysis:

- Tuberculosis
- Neoplasm
- Lung abscess
- Bronchiectasis
- Cystic fibrosis [6]

13.5 History

Care must be taken to differentiate between hemoptysis and hematemesis [6].

Hemoptysis	Hematemesis
History • Absence of nausea/vomiting • Associated hypoxia • Lung disease	History • Nausea/vomiting • Hypoxia less common • Gastrointestinal and/or hepatic disease
Sputum appearance • Frothy or clotted • Bright red or pink	Sputum appearance • Coffee ground • Dark red, brown, or black
Laboratory studies • Alkaline pH (>7)	Laboratory studies • Acidic pH (<7)

Additional pertinent historical features include:

- Amount of blood expectorated [2]
  - Mild hemoptysis: less than 30 mL in 24 h
  - Moderated hemoptysis: between 30 and 200 mL in 24 h
  - Massive hemoptysis: greater than 200 mL in 24 h
- Prior episodes of hemoptysis

  - Known parenchymal disease such as chronic obstructive pulmonary disease, recurrent pneumonia, and bronchiectasis
- Symptoms suggestive of infection (fever, chills, night sweats)
  - Pneumonia, bronchitis, upper respiratory tract infection, and sinusitis
- Weight loss
  - HIV, tuberculosis, malignancy, bronchiectasis
- Tobacco use
  - Primary lung malignancy
- Dyspnea on exertion, orthopnea, and paroxysmal nocturnal dyspnea
  - Congestive heart failure and mitral valve stenosis
- Pleuritic chest pain or recent immobilization
  - Pulmonary embolism or infarction
- Vomiting, melena, alcohol abuse, and chronic or excessive NSAID use
  - Gastric ulcer, gastric varices, Mallory-Weiss tear
- Hematuria
  - Goodpasture syndrome
- Hemoptysis associated with menses
  - Pulmonary endometriosis
- Travel history
  - Tuberculosis and fungal or parasitic infections
- Anticoagulant use
- Recent percutaneous or transbronchial procedures

13.6 Physical Examination

The physical examination may provide insight on the cause and location of the bleeding:

- Vital signs
  - Fever, hypo-/hyperthermia, and elevated respiratory rate should alert the physician to possible infectious etiology.
  - Tachycardia:
    - Appropriate fever response
    - Compensatory mechanism in maintaining perfusion in response to intravascular volume deficits and vasodilation as seen in sepsis
  - Hypoxia on pulse oximetry may be an indication of massive hemoptysis and should prompt immediate intervention.
- Head, ears, eyes, nose, and throat
  - Focus on alternative sources of bleeding.
  - Saddle nose and septal perforation should heighten suspicion for Wegener's granulomatosis [6].
  - Stridor in a child may be suggestive of aspiration of a foreign body [5].
- Cardiovascular
  - Rumbling diastolic murmur suggestive of mitral stenosis.

  - New murmur in addition to fever could suggest endocarditis with resulting septic pulmonary emboli.
  - S3 and JVD suggestive of congestive heart failure.
- Pulmonary/chest
  - Evaluate for signs of consolidation, wheezing, rales, and trauma.
- Gastrointestinal
  - Vomiting, abdominal tenderness, and ascites
- Extremities
  - Unilateral swelling may be seen with deep vein thrombosis and/or pulmonary embolus.
- Integumentary
  - Clubbing suggests lung malignancy or chronic obstructive disease.
  - Cutaneous purpura or ecchymosis may suggest a blood dyscrasia or anticoagulant use.

13.7 Diagnosis

For patients that present with hemoptysis without airway compromise, the initial evaluation of choice is chest radiography [8].

If the chest radiograph is *normal* and the patient is at risk for malignancy, computed tomography is recommended and bronchoscopy may also be considered [8].

If the chest radiograph is *abnormal*, computed tomography should be obtained to delineate the abnormality [8].

In addition, computed tomography prior to embolization can reveal the source of hemoptysis. It has also been shown that CT is more efficient than bronchoscopy in identifying the cause of bleeding [9].

13.8 Management Approaches

13.8.1 Massive Hemoptysis

Initial management entails maintaining airway patency, localizing the source, and controlling the bleeding.

In massive hemoptysis, the threat is asphyxiation, not exsanguination. If intubation is necessary, a large-bore endotracheal tube (8.5 mm in diameter or greater) is preferred in order to allow for fiber-optic evaluation. If the source is known, the patient can be placed in the lateral decubitus position toward the site of bleeding such that the blood is isolated to the bleeding lung due to gravity, leaving the non-bleeding lung fully aerated [9].

Early bronchoscopy is the procedure of choice as it facilitates localization and possible intervention. Rigid bronchoscopy is preferred as it allows for more effective suctioning [9]. If bronchoscopy is unsuccessful, interventional angiography is the next choice in therapy with bronchial artery embolization the most common approach to control bleeding [10]. These patients are typically admitted to the hospital—even in an intensive care setting. Consultation with a pulmonologist is advisable as well.

13.8.2 Non-massive Hemoptysis

A stable patient with non-massive hemoptysis should undergo initial evaluation with chest radiography. The most common cause of negative chest radiography in a patient with acute non-massive hemoptysis is bronchitis. Low-risk patients may be treated on an outpatient basis with close primary care follow-up and antibiotics if indicated [8]. If the hemoptysis persists with repeated visits or is unexplained at initial presentation, outpatient pulmonology evaluation may be needed [8]. If the imaging is abnormal, labs should be obtained with admission for further workup [11].

References

1. Khalil A, Fedida B, Parrot A, Haddad S, Fartoukh M, Carette MF. Severe hemoptysis: from diagnosis to embolization. Diagn Interv Imaging. 2015;96(7–8):775–88. https://doi-org.ezproxy.med.ucf.edu/10.1016/j.diii.2015.06.007
2. Mondoni M, Carlucci P, Job S, Parazzini EM, Cipolla G, Pagani M, Tursi F, Negri L, Fois A, Canu S, Arcadu A, Pirina P, Bonifazi M, Gasparini S, Marani S, Comel AC, Ravenna F, Dore S, Alfano F, Sferrazza Papa GF, et al. Observational, multicentre study on the epidemiology of haemoptysis. Eur Respir J. 2018;51(1):1701813. https://doi-org.ezproxy.med.ucf.edu/10.1183/13993003.01813-2017.
3. Davidson K, Shojaee S. Managing massive hemoptysis. Chest. 2020;157(1):77–88. https://doi-org.ezproxy.med.ucf.edu/10.1016/j.chest.2019.07.012.
4. Fartoukh M, Khoshnood B, Parrot A, Khalil A, Carette MF, Stoclin A, Mayaud C, Cadranel J, Ancel PY. Early prediction of in-hospital mortality of patients with hemoptysis: an approach to defining severe hemoptysis. Respiration. 2012;83(2):106–14. https://doi-org.ezproxy.med.ucf.edu/10.1159/000331501.
5. Simon DR, Aronoff SC, Del Vecchio MT. Etiologies of hemoptysis in children: a systematic review of 171 patients. Pediatr Pulmonol. 2017;52(2):255–9. https://doi-org.ezproxy.med.ucf.edu/10.1002/ppul.23497.
6. Ingbar D, Weinberger S. Etiology of hemoptysis in adults. UpToDate; 2021. http://www.uptodate.com/contents/etiology-of-hemoptysis-in-adults. Accessed 20 Sept 2022.
7. Yendamuri S. Massive airway hemorrhage. Thorac Surg Clin. 2015;25(3):255–60.
8. O'Gurek D, Choi H. Hemoptysis: evaluation and management. Am Fam Physician. 2022;105(2):144–51.
9. Radchenko C, Alraiyes A, Shojaee S. A systematic approach to the management of massive hemoptysis. J Thorac Dis. 2017;9(Suppl 10):S1069–86. https://jtd.amegroups.com/article/view/15576/12552.
10. Tom LM, Palevsky HI, Holsclaw DS, Trerotola SO, Dagli M, Mondschein JI, Stavropoulos SW, Soulen MC, Clark TW. Recurrent bleeding, survival, and longitudinal pulmonary function

following bronchial artery embolization for hemoptysis in a U.S. adult population. J Vasc Intervent Radiol. 2015;26(12):1806–13.e1. https://doi-org.ezproxy.med.ucf.edu/10.1016/j.jvir.2015.08.019.

11. Kassutto S, Weinberger S. Evaluation of nonlife-threatening hemoptysis in adults. UpToDate; 2021. http://www.uptodate.com/contents/evaluation-of-nonlife-threatening-hemoptysis-in-adults. Accessed 20 Sept 2022.

14 Abdominal Pain

Derrick Huang and Rohan Wanchu

14.1 Introduction

Abdominal pain is one of the most common complaints in the emergency department (ED), comprising approximately 5–10% of total visits [1–3]. The differential diagnosis is broad and challenging, and about a fourth of these patients seen in the ED with abdominal pain are either discharged or admitted with undifferentiated abdominal pain. This poses a challenge for both the primary care and specialist physician, as well as for the patient.

For the most part, acute and life-threatening causes of abdominal pain are addressed during the ED visit. Most patients seen in outpatient settings would either have chronic or recurrent abdominal pain or be in follow-up for acute abdominal pain. In this chapter, we will limit our discussion to chronic and recurrent abdominal pain.

14.2 Special Populations

These groups of patients may need special attention because of the broader differential diagnosis and because they may have atypical signs and symptoms of abdominal pain and thus a greater potential for serious complications [4].

14.2.1 Women

- Nonpregnant women presenting with lower abdominal pain should prompt the physician to assess for underlying pelvic disease including:
  - Infectious etiologies (i.e., sexually transmitted infections)

D. Huang (✉) · R. Wanchu
University of Central Florida, Orlando, FL, USA

B. K. Desai et al. (eds.), *Primary Care for Emergency Physicians*,
https://doi.org/10.1007/978-3-031-64676-8_14

  - Pelvic inflammatory disease
  - Acute cystitis/pyelonephritis
  - Dysmenorrhea
  - Endometriosis
  - Adenomyosis
  - Ovarian torsion
  - Ovarian cyst/rupture
  - Sexual assault or non-accidental trauma
  - Gynecological malignancies
- Pregnancy-related complications may include:
  - Ectopic pregnancies.
  - Placenta previa.
  - Vasa previa.
  - Preeclampsia.
  - Placental rupture.
  - Pregnancy should *always* be considered especially in women of the child-bearing age.
- Postmenopausal women
  - Malignancy [4]
    For example, endometrial carcinoma

14.2.2 Older Adults

- A number of older adults have underlying chronic diseases such as atherosclerosis, arthritis, and long-standing autoimmune disease, and because of the chronicity and slow progression of these chronic diseases, older patients may have atypical and very subtle signs and symptoms as compared to the younger patients [5].
- This makes the examining physician vulnerable to missing severe, life-threatening disease.
- It is important to determine the patient's risk factors and to be vigilant identifying subtle disease.
- Common serious events may include:
  - Ruptured abdominal aortic aneurysm
  - Mesenteric ischemia
    Both acute and chronic
  - Myocardial infarction
  - Intestinal obstruction
  - Malignancies

14.2.3 Immunocompromised and Immunosuppressed Patients

- Similar to older adults, these patients may also present with subtle signs and symptoms.
- Immunocompromised patients include:
  - Immune deficient
  - HIV
  - Diabetics
  - Patients on dialysis
- Immunosuppressed patients include:
  - Patients undergoing chemotherapy
  - Patients on short- or long-term immunosuppressants)

These groups of patients may not be able to illicit an appropriate response to infections or inflammation [6, 7].

14.3 Evaluation

Initial evaluation involves a thorough history and physical examination which will eventually help the examining physician determine the severity and acuteness of the disease.

- Patients that present with intense, persistent abdominal pain, extreme tenderness on exam, and features of hemodynamic instability would be concerning for an acute abdomen (i.e., appendicitis, peritonitis, mesenteric ischemia, aortic dissection, etc.) and would need emergent treatment; this might include consultation with general surgery and vascular surgery.
- Patients that present with fevers, gastrointestinal bleeding, anemia, weight loss, and signs of malnutrition or dehydration may still have an organic etiology of pain and need an urgent—not emergent—evaluation.
- A thorough physical examination should include:
  - Systolic blood pressure which generally does not decreased until 30–40% blood loss has occurred [1]. Tachycardia might develop late in the disease course.
  - Elevated temperature might point to an infectious cause; however, be aware of the patient population that might not mount a fever like the elderly or immunocompromised. Elderly patients can sometimes present with hypothermia rather than hyperthermia [8]. If there is any concern for inaccurate temperature readings, a rectal temperature should be checked.
  - The physical exam should include inspection, auscultation, and palpation.
- A pitfall is not fully examining the patient:
  - Since abdominal wall pain or examination of certain skin lesions (i.e., herpetic lesions) should be assessed during the initial visit as these conditions can be easily managed and unnecessary and expensive workup avoided.

– Many patients might be embarrassed about discussing their GU complaints and might present with more vague symptoms. A thorough GU history and physical exam when indicated is of significant importance when the chief complaint is abdominal pain especially in the pediatric and certain elderly patients who might not be able to verbalize their complaints appropriately.

Once initial evaluation has been performed and the differential diagnosis narrowed, subsequent workup may be necessary. This may potentially involve obtaining certain labs, imaging, endoscopic evaluation, and potentially even surgical procedures.

14.4 Differential Diagnosis

	Clinical features	Comment(s)
Epigastric pain		
Acute myocardial infarction	• May be associated with shortness of breath, exertional symptoms, nausea, vomiting, diaphoresis, and palpitations	• Elderly patient with risk factors for coronary artery disease • ECG may be consistent for ST elevation myocardial infarction
Acute pancreatitis	• Acute-onset, severe epigastric pain radiating to the back • Associated with nausea and vomiting	• Associated with elevated lipase acutely • If no obvious etiology, consider US • CT might be negative in the acute setting
Chronic pancreatitis	• Epigastric pain radiating to the back • Calcifications and atrophy may be seen on imaging	• Associated with pancreatic insufficiency • Some may have diabetes • Lipase may not be elevated in cases of chronic pancreatitis • CT and plain films can identify characteristic pancreatic calcifications
Mallory–Weiss tear and Boerhaave syndrome	• Mallory–Weiss: multiple episodes of vomiting leading to mucosal tears, may present with blood-tinged emesis and coffee-ground emesis • Boerhaave: crepitus on exam; pain can radiate to the back	• Mallory–Weiss is usually self-limiting and a clinical diagnosis • Boerhaave: XR can be normal in 15% of cases; gold standard is esophagogram using water-soluble contrast agent

	Clinical features	Comment(s)
Peptic ulcer disease	• Persistent, sharp stabbing pain • Usually associated with food intake, melena, and coffee-ground emesis	• Associated with NSAID use, *H. pylori* infection • Can lead to perforation and sepsis • Upright plain film can show air under the diaphragm if perforated
Gastroesophageal reflux disease	• Heartburn, usually associated with food intake • Can also occur with spasm	• Need to rule out ACS in the patient with risk factors • Improvement with GI cocktail is nondiagnostic
Gastritis/ gastropathy	• Abdominal discomfort/pain, heartburn, nausea, vomiting, and hematemesis	• Variety of etiologies including alcohol, NSAIDs, and *H. pylori*
Gastroparesis	• Nausea, vomiting, abdominal pain, early satiety, postprandial fullness, and bloating	• Most causes are idiopathic, due to diabetes, hypothyroidism, or postsurgical in nature • Seen in Parkinson's disease • Nausea and vomiting can be improved with haloperidol
Left upper quadrant pain		
Splenomegaly	• Pain may radiate to left shoulder • May have palpable spleen on examination	• Multiple etiologies • Special care in patients with sickle cell disease
Splenic infarct	• Severe LUQ pain • Splenomegaly	• Associated with hypercoagulable states and embolism, blood-borne malignancies, and blunt abdominal trauma
Splenic abscess	• Associated with fever and LUQ tenderness	• Common complication after splenic infarction
Splenic rupture	• May complain of LUQ, left chest wall, or left shoulder pain that is worse with inspiration	• Most often associated with trauma • If hemodynamically unstable and positive FAST exam requires immediate OR
Right upper quadrant pain		
Biliary colic	• Intermittent, intense, and dull discomfort	• Associated with gallbladder or biliary disease
Acute cholecystitis	• Intense pain and sometimes with fever • May have a (+) Murphy's sign	• May see pericholecystic fluid and gallstones on ultrasound

	Clinical features	Comment(s)
Acute cholangitis	• Fever, jaundice, and RUQ pain	• Associated with biliary duct infection or obstruction • Patients are typically very ill
Sphincter of Oddi dysfunction	• Intermittent biliary-type pain • May occasionally have elevated lipase and amylase	• Biliary-type pain without other apparent causes • Can be worsened with morphine
Acute hepatitis	• RUQ pain with fatigue, malaise, nausea, vomiting, and anorexia • Patients may also have jaundice	• Variety of etiologies include hepatitis A, alcohol, and drug-induced
Perihepatitis (Fitz-Hugh–Curtis syndrome)	• Pain associated with coughing or breathing • Referred pain to the right shoulder	• Usually in women with gonorrhea or chlamydia infection
Liver abscess	• Fever and abdominal pain • Transaminitis is common	• Risk factors include diabetes, underlying hepatobiliary or pancreatic disease, or liver transplant
Budd–Chiari syndrome	• Associated with signs of portal hypertension, without cirrhosis • Hepatosplenomegaly	• From occlusion of the hepatic vein
Portal vein thrombosis	• Associated with signs of portal hypertension	• Most commonly associated with cirrhosis
Lower abdominal pain		
Appendicitis	• Severe, localized RLQ pain or poorly defined umbilical pain when early on in disease course • Migration of pain to the RLQ • May have positive Rovsing and McBurney's signs; however, RLQ pain with palpation is most sensitive • Associated with leukocytosis, anorexia, and vomiting	• Emergent surgical evaluation is necessary • Usually also given IVF and antibiotics
Diverticulitis	• Constant pain, common in the LLQ (sigmoid colon)	• Inflammation of a diverticulum • CT generally not required if symptoms are consistent with last episode
Epiploic appendagitis	• Acute or subacute abdominal pain	• Benign and self-limited condition of epiploic appendages
Nephrolithiasis	• Severe flank pain but may have back, flank, or abdominal pain • Pain is usually episodic in nature	• Causes symptoms as stone passes from renal pelvis to ureter • Pain may shift from flank to groin

	Clinical features	Comment(s)
Pyelonephritis	• Associated with dysuria, frequency, urgency, hematuria, fever, chills, flank pain, and costovertebral angle tenderness	• Associated with pyuria • CT may show inflammatory stranding around the affected kidney • Can lead to abscess formation
Acute urinary retention	• Present with lower abdominal pain and discomfort; inability to urinate	• Associated with urinary obstruction • Drainage of the bladder is typically curative • Should obtain bladder scan prior to drainage
Cystitis	• Associated with dysuria, frequency, urgency, and hematuria	• Common in females • In adult males, by default it is considered a complicated cystitis
Inflammatory bowel disease	• Chronic abdominal pain, associated with diarrhea and bloody stools • Crohn's patient may have fistula formation or bowel obstruction	• May be from Crohn's disease or ulcerative colitis • Look for extraintestinal complications like uveitis, arthritis, and dermatitis
Infectious colitis	• Diarrhea as the predominant symptom but may also have associated abdominal pain, which may be severe	• Most frequently caused by *Salmonella* and *E. coli* • Usually self-limiting but certain patients may require antibiotics
Abdominal wall pain		
Abdominal wall hernias	• A small subcutaneous mass may be felt in the midline (epigastric hernia) or through the Spigelian fascia (Spigelian hernia)	• Most can be reduced unless there are signs of strangulation like peritonitis, erythema, or necrosis of the overlying skin, in which case general surgery needs to be consulted immediately
Surgical scars	• Pain around previous surgical scar, usually at the edge of the scar	• May be seen on either incisional scar or from laparoscopy (insertion point of trocar)
Abdominal wall endometriosis	• Common in women with previous Cesarean section	• Treated similarly to regular endometriosis
Radicular pain	• Disease involving T7–T12 nerve roots • Common in patient with diabetic neuropathy and spinal cord disease	• Examine the spine and back. Tricyclic drugs may be beneficial • Rule out red flags
Costochondritis	• Tenderness in the lower chest or xiphoid • Associated with nausea and even vomiting when pressure is applied to the painful site	• Most common cause of chest pain in children but can also be seen in adult women • Diagnosis of exclusion in adult population

	Clinical features	Comment(s)
Rectus sheath hematoma	• Hematoma or ecchymosis may be seen in the anterior abdomen • May have a history of trauma to the abdomen	• Common in patient with bleeding dyscrasia or on anticoagulation
Others		
Irritable bowel syndrome	• Abnormal stool frequency (≤3 bowel movements per week or >3 bowel movements per day), abnormal stool form (lumpy/hard or loose/watery), defecation straining, urgency, or a feeling of incomplete bowel movement, passing mucus and bloating	• Patients must not have rectal bleeding, nocturnal or progressive abdominal pain, weight loss, anemia, elevated inflammatory markers, or electrolyte abnormalities
Functional dyspepsia	• Postprandial fullness, early satiety, and epigastric pain or burning for the last 3 months with symptom onset at least 6 months before diagnosis and exclusion of other causes of dyspepsia with EGD and other testing	• Cause is unclear • May be associated with gastric motility and compliance, visceral hypersensitivity, *H. pylori*, altered gut microbiota, and psychosocial dysfunction
Diabetic ketoacidosis	• Polydipsia, polyuria, or decreased urine output (due to volume depletion) • Signs of dehydration • Abdominal pain and nausea/vomiting • Tachypnea (Kussmaul's breathing) • Fruity smell on breath • Ill appearance	• Most commonly in type 1 diabetes mellitus but can occur in type 2 diabetes mellitus • Identify inciting precipitant, such as medication or dietary noncompliance, infection, and cardiac or cerebral ischemia • SGLT-2 inhibitors are associated with euglycemic DKA

14.5 Physical Examination

Physical examination must always be comprehensive. Subtle behavioral signs alone may help the physician guide his/her approach to examining the patient and arriving with an accurate diagnosis.

- Vital sign assessment
  - The presence of fever should alert the physician to a possible infectious etiology.
  - Tachycardia may have multiple etiologies including:
    - An appropriate response to fever
    - The potential use of medications or drugs, including over-the-counter medications and illicit substances
    - Active pain

  - Pulse oximetry
    May alert the clinician to the presence of an underlying pulmonary pathology
- Behavior
  - Comfortable
    Benign or functional disease
  - Lethargic
    Use of narcotics, marijuana, and other sedating medications
  - Restlessness
    Associated with withdrawal symptoms
  - Guarded
    Seen in visceral disease or peritonitis.
    Laying still may indicate that the patient may have peritonitis; any movement may cause pain.
- Neurologic assessment should focus on:
  - Level of alertness
    Sedation and agitation may be associated with drugs.
  - Encephalopathy
    Underlying metabolic or drug-related issues
- Cardiovascular and pulmonary examination
  - Crackles and rales may indicate underlying pneumonia.
- Gastrointestinal examination
  - Inspection
    Inspect the skin to look for any superficial lesions that might be causing abdominal pain, for example, skin or soft tissue infection, lesions present in a dermatomal distribution, hernias, etc.
  - Auscultation
    Bowel sounds are absent in ileus and high-pitched in obstruction.
    Friction rub may be seen with splenic infarct.
  - Palpation
    Pain to light touch can be seen in peritonitis.
    Movement may worsen pain in patients with peritonitis.
  - Percussion
    Tympany signifies bowel distention.
    Dullness may signify organomegaly or mass.
    Ascites may have shifting dullness.
  - Special maneuvers (Carnett's, psoas, Murphy's, etc.)
  - Rectal/pelvic examination (rectal mass/strictures, ectopic pregnancy, salpingitis, tubo-ovarian abscess)
- GU exam, if indicated:
  - Evaluate for hernias.
  - Evaluate the scrotum in males for high riding testicle, blue dot sign, cremaster reflex, tenderness to palpation, etc.
  - If indicated, a though exam of the genitalia must be performed.

14.6 Diagnostic Workup

The diagnostic workup will necessarily be dependent upon the clinical picture of the patient. Not all tests will be of value in all patients.

In 2022, a multidisciplinary panel of experts published the Guideline for Reasonable and Appropriate Care in the Emergency Department (GRACE-2) that provides recommendations for assessment of adult patients with low-risk, recurrent, undifferentiated abdominal pain in the ED. [9] These guidelines recommend that there is insufficient evidence to recommend safe avoidance as well as routine use of repeat computed tomography (CT) of the abdominal and pelvis. If the CT abdominal and pelvis is negative, ultrasound should not be employed unless a pelvis or biliary pathology is suspected. Furthermore, screening for depression and/or anxiety is also recommended and can be performed along with the ED evaluation. Lastly, an opioid-minimizing strategy for pain control should be employed.

The panel defined recurrent abdominal pain as two or more similar episodes within 12 months, with the time elapsed between the first episode and the current episode being ≥30 days [9]. Undifferentiated was defined as no clear etiology or diagnosis from the prior workup that included a CT of the abdominal and pelvis with IV contrast, blood work including lipase and hepatic function tests, and urinalysis. Patients could not be considered low risk if they possessed the following: unstable vital signs, acute abdominal pathology on clinical examination, age less than 18 or ≥65 years, pregnancy, acute trauma within 7 days, organ transplantation or immunosuppression, abdominal surgery within 30 days, acute cancer, inflammatory bowel disease, prior bowel obstruction, and severe active psychiatric disease.

- Laboratory tests may include:
  - CBC, BMP, liver panel, and lipase
  - Antibodies (tissue transglutaminase, etc.)
  - Pregnancy test
    Mandatory for all women of childbearing age
  - Urinalysis
- Radiologic tests may include:
  - X-rays
  - CT scans
  - MRI
  - Ultrasound
- Endoscopy—typically reserved for outpatient settings, unless the patient presents with significant hematemesis and abdominal pain, in which case it becomes an urgent test:
  - EGD
  - Enteroscopy
  - Colonoscopy
  - ERCP
- Laparoscopy/surgery
  - For examination of extraluminal disease and for obtaining biopsies

- Special testing including:
  - Nuclear testing
  - Motility testing
  - Paracentesis
  - Trigger point injections

14.7 Management

Due to the wide nature of abdominal pain etiologies, management will solely depend upon the presentation of the patient. ED management will necessarily focus on the acute treatment of pain which may include modalities not typically used in the primary care setting (e.g., opioids).

- Medical
  - Pain control may include:
    - Heating pad
    - Medications including:
      - NSAIDs
      - Acetaminophen
      - Opioids
      - Muscle relaxants
  - Pain modulators
    - Tricyclic antidepressants
    - SSRIs (selective serotonin reuptake inhibitors)
    - SNRIs (serotonin–norepinephrine reuptake inhibitors)
  - Symptom relief
    - Antidiarrheals
    - Laxatives
    - Antiemetics
    - Proton pump inhibitors
    - Histamine-2 blockers
- Endoscopic
  - Celiac plexus injections
  - Endoscopic retrograde cholangiopancreatography with decompression
  - Botox injections
- Surgical
  - Placement of pain modulation devices
- Physical therapy
- Psychiatric/behavioral modalities

14.8 Disposition

After assessment and rule-out of life-threatening pathologies, many patients may remain with undifferentiated abdominal pain. Generally, if these patients, who are without acute or life-threatening pathologies, have intact oral intake, clinical improvement on reassessment, and adequate control of pain, they may be discharged if they are able to return to the ED, given strict return precautions, and recommended outpatient follow-up [10]. For abdominal pain, return precautions should include warning symptoms and signs for pathological progression of early appendicitis or small bowel obstruction, which are the two most common surgical pathologies mistakenly discharged from the ED. [10] Patients should be given clear and written instructions that address their diets and medications.

If a critical diagnosis is identified, the patient should be admitted to the appropriate service. Patients with poor follow-up and significant disease progression may also warrant admission. Older patients who might have an atypical presentation but have higher mortality and morbidity can often benefit from a period of observation with serial abdominal exams [1].

References

1. McNamara R, Dean AJ. Approach to acute abdominal pain. Emerg Med Clin North Am. 2011;29(2):159–vii. https://doi.org/10.1016/j.emc.2011.01.013.
2. Powers RD, Guertler AT. Abdominal pain in the ED: stability and change over 20 years. Am J Emerg Med. 1995;13:301.
3. Sanson TG, O'Keefe KP. Evaluation of abdominal pain in the elderly. Emerg Med Clin North Am. 1996;14:615.
4. Lewis LM, Banet GA, Blanda M, Hustey FM, Meldon SW, Gerson LW. Etiology and clinical course of abdominal pain in senior patients: a prospective, multicenter study. J Gerontol A Biol Sci Med Sci. 2005;60(8):1071–6. https://doi.org/10.1093/gerona/60.8.1071.
5. Engberding N, Wenger NK. Acute coronary syndromes in the elderly. F1000Res. 2017;6:1791. https://doi.org/10.12688/f1000research.11064.1. PMID: 29043079; PMCID: PMC5627582.
6. Thuluvath PJ, Connolly GM, Forbes A, Gazzard BG. Abdominal pain in HIV infection. Q J Med. 1991;78:275.
7. Dropulic LK, Lederman HM. Overview of infections in the immunocompromised host. Microbiol Spectr. 2016;4(4):10.1128/microbiolspec.DMIH2-0026-2016. https://doi.org/10.1128/microbiolspec.DMIH2-0026-2016. PMID: 27726779; PMCID: PMC8428766.
8. Cooper GS, Shlaes DM, Salata RA. Intraabdominal infection: differences in presentation and outcome between younger patients and the elderly. Clin Infect Dis. 1994;19(1):146–8. https://doi.org/10.1093/clinids/19.1.146.
9. Broder JS, Oliveira J E Silva L, Bellolio F, et al. Guidelines for reasonable and appropriate care in the emergency department 2 (GRACE-2): low-risk, recurrent abdominal pain in the emergency department. Acad Emerg Med. 2022;29(5):526–60. https://doi.org/10.1111/acem.14495.
10. Macaluso CR, McNamara RM. Evaluation and management of acute abdominal pain in the emergency department. Int J Gen Med. 2012;5:789–97. https://doi.org/10.2147/IJGM.S25936.

Irritable Bowel Syndrome 15

Mar'Tina Wimberly

15.1 Introduction

Irritable bowel syndrome (IBS) is the most common functional bowel disease. It is estimated to affect up to 20% of the population. It is, however, difficult to estimate prevalence, as many patients do not seek medical care and are often unrecognized or undiagnosed by physicians [1].

IBS is a clinical diagnosis characterized by abdominal pain or discomfort with altered bowel habits thought to be due to a disorder of gut-brain interaction. Multiple comorbidities are often associated with IBS such as fibromyalgia, chronic fatigue syndrome, chronic pelvic pain, and mood disorders [2].

This is a chronic, relapsing disease, associated with a significant healthcare resource use in the USA. The yearly cost of IBS is estimated at $20 billion with direct cost being highest in the initial diagnosis of the disease. It is imperative that emergency medicine physicians properly consider red flag symptoms but use judicious discretion to decrease unnecessary testing and imaging [3].

Present recommendations from the American Gastroenterological Society and American College of Gastroenterologist are to diagnose IBS without alarm features by symptom-based guidelines such as the Rome criteria. There is no pathognomonic test or symptom for IBS [2].

M. Wimberly (✉)
Department of Community Health and Family Medicine, University of Florida College of Medicine, Gainesville, FL, USA
e-mail: marrey@ufl.edu

B. K. Desai et al. (eds.), *Primary Care for Emergency Physicians*,
https://doi.org/10.1007/978-3-031-64676-8_15

15.2 Diagnostic Criteria

15.2.1 Rome IV Criteria

Recurrent abdominal pain, on average, at least 1 day per week in the last 3 months, associated with two or more of the following:

- Related to defecation
- Associated with change in stool frequency
- Associated with a change in the form (appearance) of stool

Irritable bowel syndrome is classified into the following subgroups:

- Irritable bowel syndrome constipation predominant (IBS-C)
- Irritable bowel syndrome diarrhea predominant (IBS-D)
- Irritable bowel syndrome mixed (IBS-M)

In diarrhea predominant disease, celiac testing with endomysial antibodies or tissue transglutaminase is recommended without alarm features with suspected IBS and diarrhea symptoms. It is also recommended that fecal calprotectin or fecal lactoferrin and C-reactive proteins be checked in patients to rule out inflammatory bowel disease. Age-appropriate colorectal cancer screening should be obtained in the outpatient setting [4]. Biomarkers are becoming available for diagnostic use, but their validity and clinical significance are still undetermined [5].

Although the cause of IBS is felt to be multifactorial, the following factors are felt to contribute to the disease symptomatology [2]:

- Altered pain perception
- Altered brain-gut interaction
- Increased intestinal permeability
- Visceral hypersensitivity

Risk factors for IBS [1, 2]:

- Female sex
- Lower socioeconomic status
- Peak age 20–50
- Comorbid psychiatric conditions
- History of abuse (physical, sexual, emotional)
- Psychosocial stressors
- Food intolerances
- Enteric infections

15.3 History and Physical Examination

In the emergency department, it is critical to obtain a complete history and physical to rule out other conditions. This information will allow for a confident clinical diagnosis.

Patients with IBS present to the emergency department primarily for abdominal pain. They will often present with other coexisting symptoms due to associated conditions.

It is imperative to screen for any red flags indicative of organic pathology [6, 7]:

- Anemia (cancer, IBD)
- Chronic severe diarrhea particularly with nighttime symptoms (cancer, infection, IBD)
- Family history of GI disease (cancer, IBD, celiac disease)
- Signs of bleeding (cancer, polyps, IBD, ischemic colitis)
- Fever (infection, IBD)
- Weight loss (cancer, IBD)
- Onset after age 50 (cancer)
- Palpable mass on exam (cancer)
- Elevated inflammatory markers (IBD, infection)

Any presence of red flags needs to be further evaluated to ensure proper diagnosis.

In the absence of alarm symptoms, ultrasound, endoscopy, and stool testing, which lead to increased healthcare costs, are not recommended [4, 8]. Once red flags are eliminated and preliminary labs are negative, reassurance should be provided [8].

Without alarm symptoms, appropriate workup in the emergency department includes CBC, ESR, and CRP.

15.4 Differential Diagnosis

Many symptoms of IBS are overlapping with other GI diseases [9]. It is important to screen for red flag symptoms to appropriately rule out other conditions.

Differential Diagnosis

- Carcinoid tumor
- Celiac disease
- Colorectal cancer
- Diverticular disease
- Drug use (opiates, antidepressants, calcium channel blockers)
- Gastrointestinal infection (small bowel bacterial overgrowth, *Giardia*, *Clostridium difficile*)
- Inflammatory bowel disease (IBD)
- Ischemic colitis

- Lactose intolerance
- Thyroid disease

15.5 Treatment of IBS

Once a diagnosis is made, there are several indicated treatments for IBS that can be initiated by emergency room physicians. Treatment of IBS varies on the individual and their symptoms. Treatment will usually encompass a combination of lifestyle and diet modification, medications, and behavioral interventions [2].

Therapies include:

1. Education
   - Improve understanding of disease, pathophysiology, and recurrence.
   - Establish goals of IBS therapy as control of symptoms and improvement of quality of life (not to cure all symptoms).
2. Diet modification
   - Avoid trigger foods and common inciting foods (lactose, gluten).
   - Consider low fermentable oligosaccharides, disaccharides, monosaccharaides, and polyols (FODMAP) diet.
3. Behavioral and alternative therapies
   - Cognitive behavioral therapy
   - Hypnosis
   - Biofeedback
   - Stress reduction
   - Peppermint oil
   - Acupuncture
4. Medication management should include:
   - Careful consideration of present comorbidities
   - Consideration of medication interactions and side effects
   - Starting medications at a low dose
   - Providing a short supply until a primary care physician or gastroenterologist reevaluates the patient
   - Avoiding use of narcotics, which can cause dependence and worsen IBS symptoms

15.6 Pharmacologic Treatment

Many medications are presently indicated in treatment of IBS. Treatment is guided by predominant symptoms and severity of symptoms. Symptomatic treatment can be initiated in the emergency department. Other therapies can also be initiated if symptom-based control has failed.

15.6.1 Over-the-Counter Fiber or Laxatives

Fiber and osmotic laxatives are first-line agents used to manage constipation in IBS. Long-term uses of these medications are effective and critical in symptomatic relief. These supplements should be started at low dose and titrated to desired stool consistency.

Fiber/laxatives
Psyllium or other soluble fibers
Polyethylene glycol

Pitfalls

1. Nonsoluble fiber and polyethylene glycol can worsen bloating, gas, and cramping.
2. Wheat bran should be avoided.
3. Require self-titration and adjustment if diarrhea occurs.
4. May not improve pain of IBS.
5. Cost of over-the-counter medication not covered by insurance.

15.6.2 Over-the-Counter Antidiarrheal Medications

Loperamide is the first-line agent in management of diarrhea in IBS. Other antidiarrheal medications are not presently recommended for IBS. Loperamide works in multiple mechanisms including inhibition of peristalsis, prolonging gut transit, and reduction of fecal volume [2].

Pitfalls

1. Can lead to constipation
2. May not improve pain and global symptoms of IBS
3. Cost of over-the-counter medication not covered by insurance

15.6.3 Prosecretory Agents

Two agents are presently FDA approved for IBS-C patients. Lubiprostone is a chloride channel activation increasing intestinal fluid secretion. Linaclotide and plecanatide are agents that reduce activation of visceral pain fibers [10].

FDA-approved prosecretory agents
Lubiprostone
Linaclotide
Plecanatide

Pitfalls

1. Lubiprostone can cause dose-dependent nausea and should be taken with food.
2. Linaclotide causes diarrhea and should be given 30–60 minutes prior to breakfast to limit diarrhea.
3. Costly and poor formulary coverage.

15.6.4 Antidepressants

Antidepressants are becoming more standard in care of IBS given their effects on pain perception, mood, and motility. The two classes of agents mostly used and proven to be effective are tricyclic antidepressants (TCAs) and selective serotonin reuptake inhibitors (SSRIs). These agents are recommended in moderate to severe IBS and have been shown to effectively reduce abdominal pain of IBS [11].

Antidepressants
TCAs (nortriptyline, amitriptyline)
SSRIs (citalopram, paroxetine)

Pitfalls

1. May take weeks and several dose titrations to achieve maximum effect.
2. Caution with TCA dose-dependent anticholinergic side effects (dry mouth, urinary retention, constipation, sedation, weight gain).
3. Caution with TCA-induced QT prolongation (may need EKG to assess prior to starting).
4. SSRIs can cause sexual dysfunction, agitation, nausea, drowsiness, and diarrhea.
5. Caution with use of SSRIs and other serotonergic medications that may increase risk of serotonin syndrome.

15.6.5 Antispasmodics

Antispasmodics are used as needed or prophylactically preprandial to control abdominal pain, diarrhea, bloating, and urgency. These medications provide only short-term relief, but their long-term efficacy has not been well established historically. This is achieved through smooth muscle relaxation.

Antispasmodics
Hyoscyamine
Dicyclomine
Methscopolamine

Pitfalls

1. Can worsen constipation-dominant disease
2. Caution with anticholinergic side effects (fatigue, dry mouth, dizziness)
3. Caution with sedation
4. Caution use in elderly and cognitively impaired

15.7 Medications to Avoid

Although therapeutic medication treatment is important, it is also key to avoid medications that can possibly exacerbate IBS symptoms. A risk-benefit analysis should be performed prior to use of the following over-the-counter and prescription therapies [2]:

15.7.1 Over the Counter

- Antihistamines
- Calcium
- Iron
- Magnesium
- Nonsteroidal anti-inflammatory agents
- Probiotics
- Wheat bran

15.7.2 Prescription Drugs

- Antibiotics
- Some antidepressants
- Antiparkinson medications
- Antipsychotics
- Calcium channel blockers
- Diuretics
- Metformin
- Narcotics
- Polyethylene glycol electrolyte solutions (PEG)
- Sympathomimetics

A trial of medication discontinuation may be beneficial if it is believed to be exacerbating symptoms of IBS. Patients with IBS often report multiple medication intolerances.

References

1. Sayuk GS, Gyawali CP. Irritable bowel syndrome: modern concepts and management options. Am J Med. 2015;128:817–27.
2. Lacy BE, Pimentel M, Brenner DM, et al. ACG clinical guideline: management of irritable bowel syndrome. Am J Gastroenterol. 2021;116(1):17–44.
3. Burbige EJ. Irritable bowel syndrome: diagnostic approaches in clinical practice. Clin Exp Gastroenterol. 2010;3:127–37.
4. National Institute for Health and Care Excellence. Irritable bowel syndrome in adults: diagnosis and management. (online). 2015. http://guidance.nice.org.uk/CG61.
5. Chira A, Dumitrascu DL. Serum biomarker for irritable bowel syndrome. Chijul Med. 2015;88(3):258–64.
6. Hadley SK, Gaarder SM. Treatment of irritable bowel syndrome. Am Fam Physician. 2005;72(12):2501–8.
7. Viera AJ, Hoag S, Shaughnessy J. Management of irritable bowel syndrome. Am Fam Physician. 2002;66(10):1867–75.
8. Graham L. ACG releases recommendations on the management of irritable bowel syndrome. Am Fam Physician. 2009;79(12):1108–17.
9. Wilkins T, Pepitone C, Biju A, Schade R. Diagnosis and management of IBS in adults. Am Fam Physician. 2012;86(5):419–26.
10. Black CJ, Burr NE, Camilleri M, et al. Efficacy of pharmacological therapies in patients with IBS with diarrhea or mixed stool pattern: systematic review and network meta-analysis. Gut. 2020;69(1):74–82.
11. Ford AC, Moayyedi P, Lacy BE, et al. American College of Gastroenterology monograph on the management of irritable bowel syndrome and chronic idiopathic constipation. Am J Gastroenterol. 2014;109:s2–S26c.

Bloating

16

Karyn Governale

16.1 Introduction

Bloating is a bothersome complaint that is commonly reported to physicians; it ranks second only to abdominal pain in frequency of complaints to physicians [1]. It is estimated that around 11% of the general population report frequent bloating [2], while in another study, 31% of patients met the Rome I criteria for functional bloating [3]. In fact, 90% of patients with a diagnosis of irritable bowel syndrome (IBS) will report symptoms of bloating [4]. Unfortunately, bloating is a nonspecific term that relates to the patient's subjective sensation of their abdominal distention, fullness, or excessive gas and the physician's objective determination of identifiable abdominal distention [5]. Furthermore, abdominal bloating is present in multiple functional abdominal disorders, which include both non-emergent and emergent processes. The Rome IV criteria for function abdominal bloating and distension include the following: symptoms of recurrent abdominal bloating and distension occurring at least 1 day per week; the bloating predominates over other symptoms; the symptoms must start at least 6 months prior to diagnosis and symptoms must occur at least once weekly for the past 3 months; they should not meet criteria for IBS, functional constipation, functional diarrhea, or post-prandial distress syndrome [6].

Since the natural history of bloating is poorly understood, diagnosis of this entity is sometimes difficult due to the lack of measurable parameters for assessment and grading of the symptoms. In addition, in many instances, bloating lacks a clear pathophysiologic explanation or singular management strategy. Bloating can cause significant patient distress and concern, which may prompt a subsequent presentation to the emergency department (ED). In fact, in those patients who did not have a diagnosis of irritable bowel syndrome, 75% described their symptoms as

K. Governale (✉)
Department of Community Health and Family Medicine, UF Health Shands Hospital, Gainesville, FL, USA

B. K. Desai et al. (eds.), *Primary Care for Emergency Physicians*,
https://doi.org/10.1007/978-3-031-64676-8_16

moderate to severe and 50% reduced their daily activities due to the symptoms of bloating [7].

16.2 Pathophysiology

This disorder's pathophysiology is complicated and relies on understanding many factors. These include the natural production of gas within the gastrointestinal tract (GIT), the role of gut microflora, transit time of intestinal contents, and finally, neuronal functional with the GIT [8]. Furthermore, there are different theories on bloating etiology. These range from an increase in luminal contents (ranging from fat, liquids, gas, and stool) to an impairment of abdominal emptying, to an alteration in intra-abdominal volume displacement (also known as the abdomino-phrenic theory) or increased intestinal stimuli due to the use of specific treatments or medications. These include antibiotics, probiotics, prokinetic agents, medications for spasm and gas reduction, and tricyclic antidepressants [9].

16.2.1 Intestinal Gas Production

The normal individual has approximately 100–200 cc of gas within the gastrointestinal tract, which increases after eating, especially in the colon. Stomach distention and corresponding small bowel stimulation after eating can accelerate the transit of gas; lipids, however, can cause the retention of gas, especially within the early small bowel [10, 11]. Gas production in the colon occurs mainly through bacterial metabolism, especially those foods not fully digested in the small intestine. These include sugars such as lactose and fructose. Other foods, such as legumes and complex carbohydrates, are metabolized within the colon. Additional sources of gas within the GI tract include the swallowing of air, ingestion of carbonated beverages, and acid/alkali neutralization in the upper GIT [12, 13]. Furthermore, the small intestine readily absorbs carbon dioxide, which may be promptly consumed by some colonic bacterial species that also consume hydrogen. Thus, the total amount of gas in the intestine is ever in flux due to the normal passing of flatus; healthy patients tolerate intestinal gas easily due to efficient evacuation.

Even though an excessive volume of intestinal gas has been proposed as a mechanism for bloating and distention, most studies do not support this theory [14]. Infusion of a large amount of gas into the intestinal tract of healthy volunteers produced only slight changes in abdominal girth, whereas patients with IBS show larger changes in abdominal girth even in the absence of gas infusion [15]. While it is known that increased gas volumes are present in IBS patients compared to controls, there is poor correlation between intra-abdominal gas contents and the sensation of bloating [16]. Therefore, it has been theorized that the impaired transit of gas or an abnormal distribution of gas may be more likely to be the source of the symptoms.

16.2.2 Impairment of Gas Transit

Studies have shown that patients with IBS have abnormalities in intestinal transit that may cause the symptoms of gas and bloating. Patients with IBS-related constipation have an increased prevalence of abdominal distention and bloating. Furthermore, in the study of gas infusion noted above, patients with IBS experienced more symptoms during the infusion than healthy volunteers. Similarly, in another study of IBS patients after gas infusion, 90% of IBS patients developed intestinal gas retention compared to control subjects [15]. The amount of abdominal distension correlated with gas retention in these patients. IBS patients also had impaired gas clearance from both the small intestine and the proximal (not distal) colon [17].

16.2.3 Impaired Evacuation

The ineffective evacuation of gas results in gas retention and the symptom of pain with abdominal bloating. Specific patients (especially those with IBS, constipation, and functional bloating) have difficulty effectively evacuating gas and are more likely to develop symptoms of abdominal distention [18].

16.2.4 Other Potential Causes

These include the unconscious changing of body position to a more lordotic one, abnormal abdominal- diaphragmatic reflex, in which the diaphragm of specific patients descends while the ventral muscles relax. This leads to increased abdominal girth [19] and an abnormal sensation or perception of distention [20].

16.3 Risk Factors

- Females
  - Especially during menstruation
- Younger age
- Presence of functional gastrointestinal disorder
  - Irritable bowel syndrome
  - Dyspepsia
- Higher somatic symptom checklist score
- History of cholecystectomy
  - In terms of functional bloating
- History of hysterectomy
  - In terms of functional bloating
- History of abdominal surgery
  - For organic bloating

16.4 Differential Diagnosis

- Abnormal colonic transit
- Acute or subacute bowel ischemia
- Aerophagia
- Anorexia and bulimia
- Bacterial overgrowth in the small bowel
- Celiac disease
- Changes or disturbances to colonic microflora
- Constipation
  - Acute or chronic
- Dietary
  - Increased carbohydrate intake
  - Consumption of nonabsorbable sugars
    - Sorbitol
  - Lactose intolerance
  - Intolerance to fructose
  - Sensitivity to gluten
- Disorders of the pelvic floor
- Diverticulosis
  - Small or large bowel
- Enteropathogenic infections
- Functional bloating
- Functional dyspepsia
- Gastroparesis
- Gastric outlet obstruction
- Irritable bowel syndrome
- Malabsorptive conditions
- Neoplastic disorders
- Organic causes of small bowel motility dysfunction
  - Systemic lupus erythematosus
  - Amyloidosis

16.5 History

- Neurofibromatosis
- Parkinson's disease
- Diabetes mellitus
- Scleroderma
- Thyroid disorders, especially hypothyroidism
- Muscular dystrophies

Many patients that present to the emergency department with complaints of bloating do so because of an uncomfortable sensation of the distended abdomen.

However, though bloating can cause significant patient distress, it typically represents a benign condition. Critical historical features to ascertain are:

- The time and duration of symptoms
  - Acute nature of condition
    For an acutely distended abdomen, the physician must consider a potential surgical etiology
  - Acute on chronic nature
    These patients typically have a known condition such as IBS that has caused bloating in the past, but their current presentation to ED is due to an acute deterioration
- Diet
  - Association of symptoms with specific foods including:
    Dairy products
    Fruits (fructose)
    Sucrose-containing products
    Fatty foods
    Beans
    Hx of drinking carbonated beverages
- Presence of associated gastrointestinal problems
  - Irritable bowel syndrome
  - Gastroparesis
- Presence of significant abdominal pain
  - The clinician must determine if there are palliating features, such as relief with the passage of flatus
  - Significant abdominal pain with the presence of bloating and vital sign abnormalities may be concerning for an acute surgical emergency
- Prior diagnosis of functional gastrointestinal disorders
  - Bloating is one of the most common and bothersome complaints in patients with several functional disorders, including irritable bowel syndrome, functional dyspepsia, and functional constipation [9].
- History of psychiatric conditions
  - Anxiety
  - Depression
- History of metabolic disorders
  - Diabetes mellitus
  - Hypothyroidism
- Red flag symptoms [21]
  - Blood in stool
  - Fever
  - Jaundice
  - Tenesmus
  - Dysphagia
  - Odynophagia
  - New onset symptoms in patient over 55 years of age

  - Unintentional weight loss
  - Anemia
  - Nocturnal gastrointestinal symptoms
  - Vomiting
  - All may suggest an organic or worrisome cause of bloating
- Medication history
  - May identify agents that slow gastrointestinal transit time or alter motility
- Family history may be important including:
  - History of celiac disease
  - Inflammatory bowel disease
  - Intolerance to lactose

16.6 Physical Examination

Examine the patient closely for:
- Evidence of weight loss
- Anemia
  - Conjunctival pallor, etc.
- Anxiety
- Hyperventilation with subsequent aerophagia
- Liver and spleen enlargement
- Evidence of intestinal obstruction
  - Hyperactive bowel sounds
  - Tympany on percussion
- Evidence of ascites
- Attempt to examine patient in the supine and standing positions
  - This may confirm the distention by removing exaggeration of lumbar lordosis with its consequent abdominal protuberance.

16.7 Diagnosis

Since a formal diagnosis is out of the purview of the emergency physician, the evaluation for a life- threatening process is paramount. Thus, the workup initiated in the ED for bloating will entirely depend on the clinical scenario. If the bloating is acute, an evaluation for a potential surgical etiology must be considered. If acute on chronic, typically a careful history and physical examination will elucidate the potential cause. For these conditions, appropriate follow-up will be crucial.

16.8 Introduction to Treatment

Treatment of bloating is highly individualized and typically proceeds in a stepwise fashion. First is the identification of the main symptoms: abdominal distention, bloating, or both. This may provide insight into the underlying pathophysiology of the condition. From this point, the clinician has some options, including:

16.8.1 Education

1. Dietary modifications—Those patients who ingest dairy, fructose, and fiber, for example, should be counseled to limit intake of foods with these substances since they readily ferment within the colon. Patients should be counseled to eliminate one at a time to identify the offending agent.
2. Exercise—Exercise and the limitation of recumbent periods has been shown to increase intestinal gas clearance and reduce symptoms of bloating [22].

16.8.2 Pharmacologic Treatment

Most non-prescription-based treatment options have not been well studied but may be of some benefit in specific patient population.

16.8.2.1 Over-the-Counter Medications

Simethicone is an antifoaming agent that alters the elasticity of gas bubbles and improves the passage of flatus. This has improved symptoms in some patients.

Bulking agents, including psyllium, have been used as first-line agents for patients with IBS and chronic constipation. They have been shown to decrease the frequency and severity of bloating if taken for several months.

16.8.2.2 Probiotics

These are live microorganisms that may offer a health benefit when consumed in adequate amounts. These, too, have not been studied in-depth. Some probiotics, including those with *Lactobacillus acidophilus* and *Bifidobacterium lactis,* have improved bloating severity over an 8-week period in those patients with non-constipated functional bowel disorders [23].

16.9 Introduction to Prescription Medications

Caution is urged when considering these medications and appropriate follow-up and consideration of consultation should be made prior to prescribing them.

16.9.1 Antibiotics

Rifaximin is a gut-selective antibiotic that is not absorbed systemically and has been well studied for the treatment of bloating. Patients who received this antibiotic

(400 mg three times a day for 10 days) reported improvement in both IBS symptoms and bloating compared to placebo.

16.9.2 Antispasmodics

Since these medications are used to control abdominal pain in patients with IBS, it seems intuitive that these medications may be used to treat symptoms of bloating. However, since they relax smooth muscle, they may have the potential to further cause gas accumulation in the GI tract as well as delay transit of gas through the GI tract. Therefore, their routine use is not recommended.

16.9.3 Tricyclic Antidepressants

This class of medication is used to treat functional abdominal pain and has been shown to be effective with both pain control and improvement in bloating.

16.9.3.1 Prokinetic Agents: Neostigmine

This medication is a potent cholinesterase inhibitor that is typically used while in the hospital under the supervision of a specialist, which limits its utility.

16.9.3.2 Prokinetic Agents: Metoclopramide

This medication is a dopamine antagonist approved to treat diabetic gastroparesis, as patients with this condition commonly have symptoms of bloating. This medication should be used with caution, as there are no studies that prove its benefit, and it can cause extrapyramidal symptoms and tardive dyskinesia.

16.9.4 Osmotic Laxatives

Polyethylene glycol is a nontoxic, water-soluble substance absorbed in trace amounts and approved for the short-term treatment of chronic constipation. The usage of this medication has also been shown to relieve bloating as well.

References

1. Rao SSC. Belching, bloating, and flatulence. Postgrad Med. 1997;101(4):263–9, 275–8.
2. Szarka L, Levitt M. Belching, bloating and flatulence. American College of Gastroenterology; 2006.
3. Drossman DA, Li Z, Andruzzi E, et al. U.S. householder survey of functional gastrointestinal disorders. Prevalence, sociodemography, and health impact. Dig Dis Sci. 1993;38:1569–80.
4. Houghton LA, Lea R, Agrawal A, Reilly B, Whorwell PJ. Relationship of abdominal bloating to distention in irritable bowel syndrome and effect of bowel habit. Gastroenterology. 2006;131:1003–10.

5. Azpiroz F, Malagelada JR. Abdominal bloating. Gastroenterology. 2005;129(3):1060–78.
6. Lacy BE, Cangemi D, Vazquez-Roque M. Management of chronic abdominal distension and bloating. Clin Gastroenterol Hepatol. 2021;19(2):219–231.e1. https://doi.org/10.1016/j.cgh.2020.03.056. Epub 2020 Apr 1. PMID: 32246999.
7. Sandler RS, Stewart WF, Liberman JN, Ricci JA, Zorich NL. Abdominal pain, bloating, and diarrhea in the United States: prevalence and impact. Dig Dis Sci. 2000;45:1166–71.
8. Lacy BE, Gabbard SL, Crowell MD. Pathophysiology, evaluation, and treatment of bloating: hope, hype, or hot air? Gastroenterol Hepatol. 2011;7(11):729.
9. Iovino P, Bucci C, Tremolaterra F, Santonicola A, Chiarioni G. Bloating and functional gastro-intestinal disorders: where are we and where are we going? World J Gastroenterol. 2014;20(39):14407.
10. Serra J, Azpiroz F, Malagelada JR. Gastric distension and duodenal lipid infusion modulate intestinal gas transit and tolerance in humans. Am J Gastroenterol. 2002;97:2225–30.
11. Harder H, Serra J, Azpiroz F, Malagelada JR. Reflex control of intestinal gas dynamics and tolerance in humans. Am J Physiol Gastrointest Liver Physiol. 2004;286:G89–94.
12. Levitt MD. Volume and composition of human intestinal gas determined by means of an intestinal washout technic. N Engl J Med. 1971;284:1394–8.
13. Lasser RB, Bond JH, Levitt MD. The role of intestinal gas in functional abdominal pain. N Engl J Med. 1975;293:524–6.
14. Accarino A, Perez F, Azpiroz F, Quiroga S, Malagelada JR. Intestinal gas and bloating: effect of prokinetic stimulation. Am J Gastroenterol. 2008;103:2036–42.
15. Serra J, Azpiroz F, Malagelada JR. Impaired transit and tolerance of intestinal gas in the irritable bowel syndrome. Gut. 2001;48:14–9.
16. Koide A, Yamaguchi T, Odaka T, et al. Quantitative analysis of bowel gas using plain abdominal radiograph in patients with irritable bowel syndrome. Am J Gastroenterol. 2000;95:1735–41.
17. Hernando-Harder AC, Serra J, Azpiroz F, et al. Colonic responses to gas loads in subgroups of patients with abdominal bloating. Am J Gastroenterol. 2010;105:876–82.
18. Passos MC, Serra J, Azpiroz F, Tremolaterra F, Malagelada JR. Impaired reflex control of intestinal gas transit in patients with abdominal bloating. Gut. 2005;54:344–8.
19. Accarino A, Perez F, Azpiroz F, Quiroga S, Malagelada JR. Abdominal distention results from caudo-ventral redistribution of contents. Gastroenterology. 2009;136:1544–51.
20. Bouin M, Plourde V, Boivin M, et al. Rectal distention testing in patients with irritable bowel syndrome: sensitivity, specificity, and predictive values of pain sensory thresholds. Gastroenterology. 2002;122:1771–7.
21. Wilkinson JM, Cozine E, Loftus CG. Gas, bloating, and belching: approach to evaluation management. Am Fam Physician. 2019;99(5):301–9.
22. Villoria A, Serra J, Azpiroz F, Malagelada JR. Physical activity and intestinal gas clearance in patients with bloating. Am J Gastroenterol. 2006;101:2552–7.
23. Ringel-Kulka T, Palsson OS, Maier D, et al. Probiotic bacteria Lactobacillus acidophilus NCFM and Bifidobacterium lactis bi-07 versus placebo for the symptoms of bloating in patients with functional bowel disorders: a double-blind study. J Clin Gastroenterol. 2011;45:518–25.

17 Constipation

Derrick Huang

17.1 Introduction

Constipation is a problem affecting between 12 and 19% of people within the United States [1] and is described as infrequent defecation and/or difficulty passing stool [2]. This condition is more common in certain groups including women, children, and the elderly [3]. The Rome IV diagnostic criteria define functional constipation as including two or more of the following elements occurring in at least 25% of defecations: straining, lumpy or hard stool, sensation of incomplete evacuation, sensation of anorectal obstruction/blockage, and use of manual maneuvers to facilitate defecation. Another element is experiencing fewer than three spontaneous defecations per week [4]. These elements should be present for ≥3 months with a symptom onset of ≥6 months ago. Additionally, the Rome criteria requires that loose stools are rarely present without the use of laxatives, and the patient does not meet Rome IV diagnostic criteria for irritable bowel syndrome.

17.2 Primary Constipation

- Normal transit constipation: functional constipation—most common
  - Stool passes through the colon at a normal rate.
- Slow transit constipation: prolonged delay of passage of stool through the colon [5]
  - Patients complain of abdominal bloating and infrequent bowel movements [6].
  - Theorized to be due to abnormalities of myenteric plexus, defective cholinergic innervation, and anomalies of the noradrenergic neuromuscular transmission system [5].

D. Huang (✉)
University of Central Florida, Orlando, FL, USA

B. K. Desai et al. (eds.), *Primary Care for Emergency Physicians*,
https://doi.org/10.1007/978-3-031-64676-8_17

- Anorectal dysfunction: inefficient coordination of the pelvic musculature in the evacuation mechanism [7]
  - Patients complain of feeling of incomplete emptying, sensing obstruction, or a need for digital manipulation.
  - Usually is an acquired behavioral disorder.

17.3 Secondary Constipation: Wide Array of Sources [8–10]

- **Endocrine/metabolic disorders**
  - Hyperparathyroidism
  - Diabetes mellitus
  - Uremia
  - Hypercalcemia
  - Hypothyroidism
- **Myopathic conditions**
  - Amyloidosis
  - Myotonic dystrophy
  - Scleroderma
- **Neurologic diseases**
  - Autonomic neuropathy
  - Cerebrovascular disease
  - Hirschsprung's disease
  - Multiple sclerosis
  - Parkinson's disease
  - Spinal cord injury/tumor
- **Psychological conditions**
  - Anxiety/depression
  - Somatization
- **Structural abnormalities**
  - Anal fissure/stricture or hemorrhoid
  - Colonic stricture
  - Inflammatory bowel disease
  - Obstructive colonic mass
  - Rectal prolapse or rectocele
- **Others**
  - Irritable bowel syndrome
  - Pregnancy
  - Medications

    Antacids, anticholinergics, antidepressants, antihistamines, calcium channel blockers, clonidine, diuretics, iron, levodopa, narcotics, NSAIDS, opioids, psychotropics, and sympathomimetics

17.4 Diagnosis [11]

- Primarily through history and physical examination
  - Nature and duration of constipation and drug history.
  - Assess for abdominal tenderness or distention.
  - Rectal examination may identify anal fissures and hemorrhoids which can contribute to painful defecation. Also assess anal sphincter tone for evaluation of neurological disorders which may impair sphincter function. Digital rectal exam may also reveal a rectal mass or retained stool.
- Labs
  - CBC
  - BMP: calcium and creatinine levels
  - TSH
- Endoscopy
  - Colonoscopy in patients 45 years of age or older
  - Patients with constipation and "red flag" symptoms of rectal bleeding, heme-positive stool, iron deficiency anemia, weight loss of >10 lbs, obstructive symptoms, or family history of colorectal cancer
- Imaging: radiography not especially helpful but may detect stool retention
  - Barium radiographs may help detect Hirschsprung's disease.
- Secondary tests such as anorectal manometry and colonic transit studies can be helpful in evaluation of patients whose constipation is refractory to initial treatment measures.

17.5 Treatment

- Nonpharmacologic treatments [12]
  - Bowel training: encourage patients to attempt defecation in the morning, shortly after awakening, when the bowels are more active, and 30 min after meals to use the gastrocolic reflex.
  - Dietary fiber intake: recommended 20–35 g daily—increase by 5 g daily until reached daily recommended intake. Increase fiber-rich foods: bran, fruits, vegetables, nuts, and prune juice [9]. Psyllium and methylcellulose are the most effective forms of fiber replacement.
- Fluid intake: decreased intake may result in fecal impaction [13].
- Regular exercise.
  - Biofeedback/pelvic floor retraining: useful for anorectal dysfunction.
- Pharmacologic treatment [14]
  - **Bulk laxatives**: Citrucel, FiberCon, and Metamucil absorb water from the intestinal lumen to increase stool mass and soften stool consistency.

    Work best for patients with functional normal transit constipation.

    Improve symptoms of constipation such as stool consistency and abdominal pain.

    Side effects include bloating and increased gas production.

– **Emollient laxatives**—stool softeners: docusate lowers surface tension, thereby allowing water to more easily enter the bowel.

Not as effective as bulk laxatives but useful in patients with painful defecation conditions such as hemorrhoids or anal fissures.

– **Osmotic laxatives**: milk of magnesia, magnesium citrate, MiraLAX, and lactulose hyperosmolar agents which use osmotic activity to result in secretion of water into the intestinal lumen.

Monitor for electrolyte imbalances such as hypokalemia and hypermagnesemia.

Use with caution in congestive heart failure and chronic renal insufficiency patients.

– **Stimulant laxatives**: Dulcolax, senna, tegaserod, castor oil, and bisacodyl increase intestinal motility and secretion of water into the bowel.

May cause abdominal cramping as a result of increased peristalsis.

Do not use in patients with suspected bowel obstruction.

References

1. Higgins PD, Johanson JF. Epidemiology of constipation in North America: a systematic review. Am J Gastroenterol. 2004;99:750–9.
2. American College of Gastroenterology Chronic Constipation Task Force. An evidence-based approach to the management of chronic constipation in North America. Am J Gastroenterol. 2005;100(Suppl 1):S1–4.
3. Lindsley CW. The top prescription drugs of 2011 in the United States: antipsychotics and antidepressants once again lead CNS therapeutics. ACS Chem Neurosci. 2012;3:630–1.
4. Longstreth GF, Thompson WG, Chey WD, et al. Functional bowel disorders. Gastroenterology. 2006;130:1480–91.
5. Rao SS. Constipation: evaluation and treatment. Gastroenterol Clin North Am. 2003;32:659–83.
6. Koch A, Voderholzer WA, Klauser AG, Muller-Lissner S. Symptoms in chronic constipation. Dis Colon Rectum. 1997;40:902–6.
7. Rao SS, Welcher KD, Leistikow JS. Obstructive defecation: a failure of rectoanal coordination. Am J Gastroenterol. 1998;93:1042–50.
8. Prather CM, Ortiz-Camacho CP. Evaluation and treatment of constipation and fecal impaction in adults. Mayo Clin Proc. 1998;73:881–6.
9. Thomas DR, Forrester L, Gloth MF, Gruber J, Krause RA, Prather C, et al. Clinical consensus: the constipation crisis in long-term care. Ann Long-Term Care. 2003;Suppl:3–14.
10. Schiller LR. Constipation and fecal incontinence in the elderly. Gastroenterol Clin North Am. 2001;30:497–515.
11. Locke GR III, Pemberton JH, Phillips SF. American Gastroenterological Association medical position statement: guidelines on constipation. Gastroenterology. 2000;119:1761–6.
12. Rao SS, Sadeghi P, Beaty J, Kavlock R, Ackerson K. Ambulatory 24-h colonic manometry in healthy humans. Am J Physiol Gastrointest Liver Physiol. 2001;280:G629–39.
13. Wrenn K. Fecal impaction. N Engl J Med. 1989;321:658–62.
14. Hsieh C. Treatment of constipation in older adults. Am Fam Physician. 2005;72:2277–84, 2285.

Diarrhea

18

Bryson Renouard

18.1 Introduction

Diarrhea is a common problem which results in nearly a million hospitalizations and 6000 deaths per year in the USA alone [1]. Diarrheal diseases are also a significant worldwide public health issue due to contaminated water and food supplies in resource-limited countries. As a result, these diseases contribute to significant morbidity and mortality rates in these regions, especially in young children.

Acute diarrhea can be defined as an increase in stool frequency up to three more times per day or greater than 200 g of stool per day for up to 14 days [2]. Subacute and chronic diarrhea are defined as diarrhea lasting from 14 to 30 days, respectively.

18.1.1 Pathophysiology

Diarrheal disease can be divided into two distinct categories: inflammatory- and noninflammatory-associated conditions. Inflammatory etiologies are typically caused by invasive pathogens or are toxin-induced, whereas noninflammatory diarrhea is typically viral but can also be caused by parasites. Inflammatory syndromes may cause mucosal disruption and result in more severe abdominal pain, blood in stool, and fever. They will also typically present with fecal leukocytes on stool evaluation. Noninflammatory conditions typically cause increased secretion into the bowel lumen resulting in more profuse, non-bloody, watery diarrhea. These patients may have abdominal cramping, but it is not typically as severe and may also present with nausea and vomiting. Noninflammatory syndromes are typically milder in nature than inflammatory syndromes.

B. Renouard (✉)
Texas A&M University, College Station, TX, USA

B. K. Desai et al. (eds.), *Primary Care for Emergency Physicians*,
https://doi.org/10.1007/978-3-031-64676-8_18

18.2 Risk Factors for Diarrhea

- Extremes of age
  - Elderly
  - Infants
- Travel
- Immunosuppressed
  - HIV
  - Chronic steroid medication use
  - Chemotherapy
- Close contact in an environment with other potentially ill people
  - Day care
  - Cruise ships
  - Military
- Exposure to contaminated food or water
- Exposure to inadequate sewage disposal
- Significant medical history of:
  - Gastrointestinal disease
    - Irritable bowel syndrome
    - Crohn's disease
    - Ulcerative colitis
    - Mesenteric ischemia
    - Colorectal cancer
    - Malabsorption
    - Short bowel syndrome
    - Bowel obstruction
    - Overflow incontinence secondary to chronic constipation
    - Lactose intolerance
    - Celiac disease
  - Endocrine disease
    - Diabetes mellitus
    - Adrenocortical insufficiency
    - Hyperthyroidism
    - Carcinoid tumor
- Medications and drugs
  - Antibiotics
  - Anti-inflammatory agents
    - NSAIDs
  - Magnesium-containing medications
    - Antacids
  - Alcohol
  - Chemotherapy
  - Colchicine
  - Laxatives
  - Others—less common

ACE inhibitors
Cholesterol-lowering medications
Lithium
Proton pump inhibitors
- Pregnancy
- Fecal-oral sexual contact

18.3 Differential Diagnosis

Since the differential diagnosis of diarrhea is extremely broad, only representative examples have been listed.

18.3.1 Acute

- Infectious diarrhea
  - Viral—majority of acute diarrheal illness
    - Rotavirus
      - Incidence has decreased with adoption of the rotavirus vaccine.
    - Norovirus
      - Implicated in many cruise ship outbreaks
  - Bacterial
    - *Salmonella*
    - *Shigella*
    - *E. coli* O157:H7
    - *Vibrio*
    - *Yersinia*
    - *Listeria*
    - *Clostridium difficile*
      - Often antibiotic induced
        - Antibiotics can alter gut flora allowing *C. difficile* to propagate.
    - Bacterial cultures are positive in only 1–5% of cases [3].
  - Protozoal
    - Giardia
      - Consumption of untreated water
  - Fungal—less common
- Foodborne illness with representative examples
  - Raw or undercooked beef
    - Shiga toxin-producing *E. coli*
    - *Staphylococcus aureus*
    - *Clostridium perfringens*
    - *Salmonella*
    - *Listeria*
    - *Bacillus cereus*

Yersinia
- Undercooked pork
  Staphylococcus aureus
  Clostridium perfringens
  Salmonella
  Listeria
  Shiga toxin-producing *E. coli*
  Bacillus cereus
  Yersinia
- Undercooked poultry
  Staphylococcus aureus
  Clostridium perfringens
  Salmonella
  Listeria
  Campylobacter
- Fried rice
  Bacillus cereus
- Seafood, including raw shellfish
  Vibrio parahaemolyticus
  Vibrio cholerae
- Raw milk
  Listeria
  Shiga toxin-producing *E. coli*
  Salmonella
  Campylobacter

- Fecal-oral sexual contact
  - *Salmonella*
  - *Shigella*
  - *Campylobacter*
  - Protozoal disease
- Day care
  - Rotavirus
  - *Shigella*
  - *Cryptosporidium*
- Medication-induced
  - *See above.*
- Travel to endemic country
  - Most common is enterotoxigenic *E. coli*.

18.3.2 Chronic

- HIV infection or immunosuppression (may be acute as well)
  - *Isospora*
  - *Listeria*

- *Mycobacterium avium-intracellulare* complex
    - *Cryptosporidium*
    - CMV
- Pregnancy
    - *Listeria*
- Alcohol abuse
- Irritable bowel syndrome
    - The most common cause of functional diarrhea in the developed world
- Malabsorption of bile acids
- Malabsorption of carbohydrates
- Celiac disease
- Crohn's disease
- Ulcerative colitis
- Congenital syndromes
- Neuroendocrine tumors
- Gastric bypass
- Mesenteric ischemia
- Short bowel syndrome
- Tropical sprue
- Whipple's disease
- Hepatobiliary disorders
- Pancreatic exocrine insufficiency
- Neoplasia
    - Colon cancer
    - Lymphoma
- Radiation colitis

18.3.3 Common Complaints and Red Flags of Acute Diarrhea

- Acute abdominal pain
    - Typically crampy in nature and benign.
    - Severe pain or pain out of proportion to the clinical picture requires a more thorough investigation.
    - Can typically present with any etiology of diarrhea.
- Acute rectal pain or signs/symptoms of proctitis
    - Syphilis
    - Gonorrhea
    - Chlamydia
    - Herpes simplex virus
    - Other etiologies include:
        - *Salmonella*
        - *Shigella*
        - *E. histolytica*
- Fever

  - Typically associated with moderate to severe diarrhea of an invasive pathogen
  - May also be associated with bloody diarrhea
  - Etiologies include:
    - *Salmonella*
    - *Shigella*
    - *Campylobacter*
    - *Yersinia*
- Nausea and vomiting
  - Often occurs with "traveler's" diarrhea
  - Etiologies include:
    - Toxin-based etiologies
      - Enterotoxigenic *E. coli*
    - *Salmonella*
    - *Campylobacter*
    - *Vibrio*
    - Viral-based etiologies
      - Rotavirus
      - Norovirus
- Bloody stools
  - Etiologies include:
    - *Salmonella*
    - *Shigella*
    - *Campylobacter*
    - *Yersinia*
    - Shiga toxin-producing *E. coli*
      - Classically has abdominal pain with no fever
- "Rice-water stools"
  - *Vibrio cholerae*
- Diarrhea with a potentially common exposure source
  - Within 6 h
    - *Staphylococcus*
    - *Bacillus cereus*
      - May have vomiting
  - After 8 h
    - *Clostridium perfringens*

18.4 Common Complaints and Red Flags of Chronic Diarrhea

- Watery, fatty stools
  - Typical of malabsorptive causes
- Bloody, pustular stools (may be intermittent for weeks-months, as opposed to several days for acute diarrhea)
  - Typical of inflammatory causes
- Important to recognize categories may overlap

- Weight loss
- Lymphadenopathy

18.5 History

When assessing a patient with a diarrheal illness, a careful history and physical is paramount in determining potential etiology of the illness. In addition to a review of medical and surgical history, specific questions that should be asked include:

- What is the usual frequency and consistency of bowel movements?
- What is the current frequency and consistency of bowel movements?
- Is there blood or mucus in the stool?
- Have there been changes to diet?
  - Any over-the-counter supplements?
- Has there been recent travel?
- What foods worsen the diarrhea?
  - Dairy products
  - Fatty foods
- Are there any new medications?
- Is the patient pregnant?
  - Concern for *Listeria* which may prompt further consultation with obstetrics
- Are there sick contacts?
- Has there been a documented fever or associated nausea and vomiting?

18.6 Physical Examination

The physical examination should focus on potential emergency conditions for the reported diarrhea and specifically for evidence of severe dehydration or sepsis.

- Vital signs and general assessment
  - The presence of fever should alert the physician to a possible infectious or inflammatory etiology.
  - Orthostatic vital signs:
    - Abnormalities also may indicate dehydration status.
  - Tachycardia may have multiple etiologies including:
    - An appropriate response to fever
    - Dehydration
  - An abnormal respiratory pattern may also be indicative of severe dehydration [4].
  - Evidence of weight loss:
    - Typically associated with chronic diarrhea.
    - Consider malignancy in this population.
  - Skin findings:
    - Jaundice

Hepatobiliary disorders
Dermatitis herpetiformis [5]
An itchy, blistering rash present in 15–25% of patients with celiac disease
Evaluation of skin turgor
Decreased turgor is another sign of dehydration.

- Neurologic assessment
  - Level of alertness
    Patients at the extremes of age may have lethargy and obtundation or even be comatose depending on the degree of illness.
- Head, eyes, ears, nose, and throat examination
  - Evidence of dehydration
    Mucus membrane moistness
    Sunken eyes
  - Evidence of episcleritis
    May be associated with inflammatory bowel disorders
- Cardiovascular and pulmonary examination
  - Note capillary refill time:
    Delayed capillary refill may indicate dehydration and decreased peripheral perfusion.
- Gastrointestinal examination [6]
  - Exposure of the abdomen is important to assess for:
    Evidence of surgical scars
    Evidence of bloating or ascites
  - Assess abdominal tenderness to palpation:
    Evaluate for a surgical etiology.
  - Assess for evidence of masses:
    Neoplasia
  - Assess bowel sounds:
    Hyperactive bowel sounds may indicate hypermotility.
  - Rectal examination is important to assess for:
    Evidence of fistula
    Crohn's disease
    Fecal occult blood testing
  - Consider anoscopy if available:
    May detect impacted stools which may be the cause of paradoxical diarrhea which is stool leakage around the impacted stool
    May detect ulcerations

18.7 Diagnostic Testing

Since most diarrhea is of a watery, benign nature, diagnostic testing is rarely required and is typically reserved for those patients who present with a more severe clinical picture, including moderate to profound dehydration, fever, bloody stools, or a significant past medical history (HIV, immunosuppression, uncontrolled diabetes mellitus, etc.).

18.7.1 Specific Tests

1. Fecal occult blood testing
   (a) A rapid and inexpensive test—utility is improved when used in combination with a positive stool lactoferrin or stool leukocyte test. If these are positive, the likelihood for an inflammatory diarrhea is more common [1].
   (b) A pitfall of fecal occult blood testing is overreliance on the test, since its sensitivity and specificity are only 71% and 79%, respectively [7].
2. Lactoferrin and leukocytes
   (a) A pitfall of stool leukocyte testing is the lack of standardization of laboratory interpretation. Coupled with the potential difficulty in handling specimens and the wide variability and sensitivity and specificity, this test has limited utility [8].
   (b) Lactoferrin is a more sensitive and specific method for assessment since it is a marker for leukocytes that is present when cells are damaged. It increases in the setting of bacterial infections [9]. It has replaced fecal leukocytes as the ideal method for the screening of leukocytes when indicated [10].
3. Stool cultures
   (a) A pitfall of stool cultures is overreliance on the test. Stool culture in every case of diarrhea is expensive and not helpful in the emergency department. However, obtaining stool cultures in those patients who have tests revealing the presence of leukocytes or who have grossly bloody stools increases the likelihood of a positive result [11].
   (b) Typically, stool cultures should be reserved for those patients who present with a severe clinical picture, including those with significant dehydration, grossly bloody stools, signs or symptoms of an inflammatory disease, prolonged symptoms (3–7 days), or a history of immunosuppression (cancer, HIV) [12].
4. Testing for ova and parasites
   (a) Like stool cultures, it is expensive and inefficient for those patients presenting the ED without historical features that warrant testing.
   (b) Historical features that *do* warrant testing include [13]:
      - Persistent diarrhea of a weeks' duration
      - Travel and/or camping in mountainous regions
        – Drinking untreated water in those areas
      - Infants in a day care setting
      - Patients with AIDS
      - Men who have intercourse with men
      - Bloody diarrhea with a lack of fecal leukocytes
      - Diarrheal outbreaks in the community
5. Testing for *Clostridium difficile*
   (a) Routine testing for *C. difficile* toxins is not indicated unless [14, 15]:
      - The patient has unexplained diarrhea after 3 days of hospitalization.
      - The patient is presently on antibiotics.
      - Diarrhea is present 1 month after antibiotic discontinuation.

   - Consideration of *C. difficile* should also be made 2–3 months after the discontinuation of antibiotics.
   - The patient has significant comorbidities as detailed previously.
6. Routine blood and urine testing
   (a) Used on a case-by-case basis to evaluate for specific abnormalities.
   (b) K+, BUN/creatinine ratio, and urine specific gravity assessment may be of benefit.
   (c) A complete blood count, albumin level, erythrocyte sedimentation rate, liver function testing, and thyroid-stimulating hormone level may be of benefit especially in chronic diarrhea.
      - Evidence of iron deficiency anemia may indicate celiac disease.
7. Other tests
   (a) Endoscopy
      - Of limited utility in the emergency department
      - May be considered by primary care providers if the diagnosis is not clear after treatment, for persistent symptoms with unremarkable blood and stool tests
      - May be of more benefit in chronic diarrheal states and the diagnosis of noninfectious etiologies of acute diarrhea (e.g., inflammatory bowel disease, cancer, etc.)
   (b) Computed tomography (CT)
      - Of little benefit in those patients with mild diarrhea and unremarkable vital signs; may be helpful in patients who have concomitant abdominal pain.
      - Of greater utility in those patients in which an underlying surgical emergency is considered (e.g., obstruction).
      - CT should be also considered if the clinician suspects an underlying significant GI bleed.

18.8 Introduction to Treatment

The initial stabilization begins with the assessment of airway, breathing, and circulation. The physician must simultaneously manage volume resuscitation with diagnostic modalities in order to determine the medical or potential surgical cause of the diarrhea.

- Rehydration
  - Emergent rehydration is a priority of the emergency physician.
  - Oral rehydration is typically preferable to intravenous solutions:

    Pitfall: May be difficult to adequately provide ongoing oral rehydration to patients in the ED.

    If given, oral rehydration should have a mixture of salt and glucose with a reduced osmolarity.

This decreases output of stool and frequency of emesis and has been shown to decrease the need for intravenous hydration [16]

It also does not increase hyponatremia [17].

A solution that the emergency physician can prescribe when sending patients home consists of ½ teaspoon of salt, 6 teaspoons of sugar, and 1 L of water.

This is strong enough to replace the electrolyte loss but not overwhelm the bowels with a hyperosmolar solution which may worsen the diarrhea.

- The best options for the rehydration of children at home are Pedialyte, Gatorade, Enfalyte, or the World Health Organization oral rehydrating solution.
- If oral rehydration is not feasible, intravenous hydration is required.
- Pitfalls
- The use of high-sugar drinks such as fruit juices or sodas will potentially worsen diarrhea and should not be used.
- "Clear" liquids (e.g., water, chicken broth) should not be used as well since they are hypoosmolar and are inadequate for the replacement of sodium, potassium, and bicarbonate.
- May potentially cause hyponatremia.

• Early feeding
  - Early feeding decreases the permeability of the intestines that is caused by infection, typically improves overall nutrition in diarrheal states, and decreases the duration of illness [18].
  - Pitfall: The commonly used "BRAT" (bananas, rice, applesauce, and toast) diet has limited evidence to support its routine use [19].
  - Pitfall: Patients typically are instructed to avoid solid foods for 24 h; this also is not helpful [20].

• Prevention
  - Factors that are important for the prevention of diarrheal illness include proper handwashing, overall good hygiene, and access to clean water.

18.9 Pharmacologic Treatment

There are several medications for the emergency physician to consider, but care must be taken to choose those medications that will have a benefit.

18.9.1 Antibiotics

Since most diarrhea is viral and typically self-limited, routine antibiotic use is not indicated for those with watery diarrhea and who are not ill-appearing on assessment. A common pitfall is the inappropriate prescribing of antibiotics which may lead to several consequences. First, the eradication of normal gut flora may lead to colonization with *C. difficile* which in turn may prolong the disease. In addition, antibiotics may lead to the delay in the excretion of organisms such as *Salmonella*, thus potentially causing a carrier state. Furthermore, the production of certain toxins, including Shiga toxins produced by organisms such as Shiga toxin-producing *E. coli*, may be enhanced. In this case, there is an increased risk of hemolytic uremic syndrome. Finally, long-term consequences of inappropriate antibiotic administration also include potential development of antibiotic resistance.

Consideration of antibiotic use should be made for those patients who are immunocompromised, those who have severe illness, including sepsis, and those patients older than 65 years of age. Diarrhea lasting for 10–14 days or greater warrants testing and potential treatment for nonviral etiologies.

Specific therapy is listed in Table 18.1.

Table 18.1 Antibiotic choices for specific bacterial agents

Agent	Brief clinical tidbits	Treatment
Campylobacter, Shigella, Salmonella, and Yersinia	Invasive diarrhea characterized by fever and bloody stools	TMP/SMX or fluoroquinolone for 3 days (may reduce duration of shedding); see below for more information regarding *Campylobacter*
Enterotoxigenic *E. coli*, *Campylobacter*, *Salmonella, Shigella, Aeromonas, Vibrio,* and *Bacteroides*	Traveler's diarrhea: watery diarrhea, +abdominal cramps, N/V, and tenesmus	TMP/SMX or fluoroquinolone for 3 days may reduce duration of illness by 2–3 days
Shigella	Severe dysentery with fever and bloody diarrhea	TMP/SMX or fluoroquinolone two times a day for 3 days
Vibrio cholerae	"Rice-water stools" and severe diarrhea	Doxycycline 300 mg × one dose or TMP/SMX two times a day for 3 days or fluoroquinolone × one dose
Campylobacter	Associated with Guillain-Barre, inflammatory bowel disease and reactive arthritis. Causes acute watery diarrhea	Azithromycin 500 mg a day for 3 days
Salmonella	Treat specific patient populations (see below)	TMP/SMX or fluoroquinolone two times a day for 5–7 days
Listeria	Treat specific patient populations (see below)	Ampicillin
C. difficile	See below	Metronidazole 500 mg orally three times a day for 10–14 days or vancomycin 125 mg orally four times a day for 10–14 days

TMP-SMX trimethoprim/sulfamethoxazole

Note: From "Diarrhea" by Desai B and Desai A, 2017, *Primary Care for Emergency Physicians*, p. 201. Copyright 2017 by Springer International Publishing Switzerland

Pitfalls

1. Treating patients who have bloody diarrhea with abdominal pain, no fever, and relevant history of eating raw ground beef or seed sprouts, with antibiotics:
   (a) There is a risk of hemolytic-uremic syndrome.
   (b) Treatment with antibiotics does not improve O157 illness.
2. Treatment of *Yersinia.* These patients present with "pseudoappendicitis" with right lower quadrant abdominal pain along with the watery diarrhea. Treatment is only required for immunocompromised patients.
3. Routine treatment of *Salmonella.* These patients may present acutely ill with fever, muscle aches, and pains, and it typically is human-to-human transmission. Treatment is recommended for those patients who are:
   (a) Immunocompromised
   (b) Are at the extremes of age
   (c) Have persistent, severe diarrhea
   (d) Have severe illness, including sepsis
   (e) Have a history of valvular heart disease
4. Routine treatment of *Listeria.* Unless pregnant or immunocompromised—in which case the disease may be severe—patients typically have mild systemic symptoms.

18.9.2 Treatment of Clostridium difficile

This organism deserves special mention as it is one of the more serious causes of diarrhea affecting patients. Prior antibiotic use (including fluoroquinolones, clindamycin, penicillins, and cephalosporins) eliminates normal gut flora allowing for colonization by *C. difficile*. The diarrhea caused by *C. difficile* is severe, with up to 15 bowel movements per day with associated abdominal pain and cramping. Many patients may have a systemic reaction, with fever, tachycardia, and tachypnea depending on level of dehydration and overall illness. Complications of *C. difficile* infection include toxic megacolon, which is an abnormal dilation of the colon that is seen on imaging studies. Those patients who do not respond to medical management may require urgent surgical consultation due to the high risk of perforation (Table 18.2).

18.9.3 Antidiarrheal Agents

Antimotility agents that are readily available over the counter, such as loperamide, may reduce the duration of diarrhea by 24 h, for those patients with non-bloody stools. In those patients with a diagnosis of traveler's diarrhea, an increased chance of cure may be obtained at 1–2 days in conjunction with antibiotics [21]. Loperamide in combination with simethicone has been shown to be of benefit in acute nonspecific diarrhea associated with intestinal gas-related discomfort compared with either

Table 18.2 Antibiotic choices for specific protozoal agents

Agent	Brief clinical tidbits	Treatment
Giardia	Persistent diarrhea after exposure to untreated water; relapses may occur due to misdiagnosis	Metronidazole 750 mg three times a day for 7–10 days
Entamoeba histolytica	Severe disease may result in hepatic abscess	Metronidazole 750 mg three times a day for 5–10 days in addition to paromomycin 25–35 mg/kg in three divided doses for 5–10 days
Cryptosporidium	Therapy may be required in immunosuppressed patients but may not be necessary in immunocompetent patients with mild disease and those patients with HIV who have a CD4 count >150 cells/mm^3	Nitazoxanide 500 mg two times a day for 3 days for severe disease
Cyclospora or *Isospora*	Requires longer therapy in HIV or immunosuppressed	TMP/SMX two times per day for 7–10 days (two to four times per day for 10–14 days for HIV or immunosuppressed)
Microsporidia	In patients with AIDS, highly active retroviral therapy may be adequate to eradicate intestinal disease	Albendazole 400 mg two times per day for 3 weeks

Note: From "Diarrhea" by Desai B and Desai A, 2017, *Primary Care for Emergency Physicians*, p. 202. Copyright 2017 by Springer International Publishing Switzerland

alone [22]. Bismuth subsalicylate is an effective alternative in patients with a fever and bloody diarrhea. It significantly reduces the number of unformed stools and improves symptoms [23].

Some antidiarrheal agents
Loperamide
Loperamide/simethicone
Bismuth subsalicylate

Pitfalls

1. Use of loperamide in bloody or potentially invasive/inflammatory diarrhea. This may prolong the duration of the illness and cause worsening of the patient's condition.

18.9.4 Probiotics

This class of over-the-counter medication is believed to work by immune system stimulation and competition for binding on the epithelial cells of the intestine. The use of probiotics in children has shown to reduce duration and severity of diarrhea by up to 1 day.

Pitfalls

1. Different strains of probiotics may have different clinical effects.

18.9.5 Zinc

Zinc has been shown in studies done in China that it too may reduce the duration of diarrhea in children less than 5 years of age. These studies showed a reduction in morbidity as a result of zinc supplementation for patients less than 5 [24]. The World Health Organization supports zinc treatment of diarrhea in low- to middle-income countries.

Pitfalls of Anticipatory Guidance

1. Providing guidance for all patients who present to the ED is paramount for their understanding of the diarrheal disease process.
2. Patients must be informed that this process may take from 3–5 days to fully run its course.
3. Return precautions of fever, bloody diarrhea, signs of significant dehydration (e.g., decrease in urine output), and lethargy should be provided.
4. Instructions on proper handwashing and good hygiene should be given.

References

1. Thielman NM, Guerrant RL. Acute infectious diarrhea. N Engl J Med. 2004;350:38–47.
2. Scallan E, Hoekstra RM, Angulo FJ, et al. Foodborne illness acquired in the United States. Emerg Infect Dis. 2011;17(1):7–15.
3. Guerrant RL, Van Gilder T, Steiner TS, et al. Practice guidelines for the management of infectious diarrhea. Clin Infect Dis. 2001;32:331–50.
4. Steiner MJ, DeWalt DA, Byerley JS. Is this child dehydrated? JAMA. 2004;291(22):2746–54.
5. Rodrigo L. Celiac disease. World J Gastroenterol. 2006;12(41):6585–93.
6. Guerrant RL, Van Gilder T, Steiner TS, et al.; Infectious Diseases Society of America. Practice guidelines for the management of infectious diarrhea. Clin Infect Dis. 2001;32(3):331–351.
7. Ilnyckyj A. Clinical evaluation and management of acute infectious diarrhea in adults. Gastroenterol Clin North Am. 2001;30(3):599–609.
8. Gill CJ, Lau J, Gorbach SL, Hamer DH. Diagnostic accuracy of stool assays for inflammatory bacterial gastroenteritis in developed and resource-poor countries. Clin Infect Dis. 2003;37(3):365–75.
9. Chen CC, Chang CJ, Lin TY, Lai MW, Chao HC, Kong MS. Usefulness of fecal lactoferrin in predicting and monitoring the clinical severity of infectious diarrhea. World J Gastroenterol. 2011;17(37):4218–24.
10. Hayakawa T, Jin CX, Ko SB, Kitagawa M, Ishiguro H. Lactoferrin in gastrointestinal disease. Intern Med. 2009;48(15):1251–4.
11. Talan D, Moran GJ, Newdow M, et al.; EMERGEncy ID NET Study Group. Etiology of bloody diarrhea among patients presenting to United States emergency departments: prevalence of *Escherichia coli* O157:H7 and other enteropathogens. Clin Infect Dis. 2001;32(4):573–580.

12. Bauer TM, Lalvani A, Fehrenbach J, et al. Derivation and validation of guidelines for stool cultures for enteropathogenic bacteria other than *Clostridium difficile* in hospitalized adults. JAMA. 2001;285(3):313–9.
13. DuPont HL. Guidelines on acute infectious diarrhea in adults. The practice parameters Committee of the American College of Gastroenterology. Am J Gastroenterol. 1997;92(11):1962–75.
14. Centers for Disease Control and Prevention. Vital signs: preventing *Clostridium difficile* infections. MMWR Morb Mortal Wkly Rep. 2012;61(9):157–62.
15. Siegel DL, Edelstein PH, Nachamkin I. Inappropriate testing for diarrheal diseases in the hospital. JAMA. 1990;263(7):979–82.
16. Hahn S, Kim Y, Garner P. Reduced osmolarity oral rehydration solution for treating dehydration due to diarrhoea in children: systematic review. BMJ. 2001;323(7304):81–5.
17. Alam NH, Yunus M, Faruque AS, et al. Symptomatic hyponatremia during treatment of dehydrating diarrheal disease with reduced osmolarity oral rehydration solution. JAMA. 2006;296(5):567–73.
18. Duggan C, Nurko S. "Feeding the gut": the scientific basis for continued enteral nutrition during acute diarrhea. J Pediatr. 1997;131(6):801–8.
19. Gadewar S, Fasano A. Current concepts in the evaluation, diagnosis and management of acute infectious diarrhea. Curr Opin Pharmacol. 2005;5(6):559–65.
20. De Bruyn G. Diarrhea in adults (acute). Am Fam Physician. 2008;78(4):503–4.
21. Riddle MS, Arnold S, Tribble DR. Effect of adjunctive loperamide in combination with antibiotics on treatment outcomes in traveler's diarrhea: a systematic review and meta-analysis. Clin Infect Dis. 2008;47(8):1007–14.
22. Hanauer SB, DuPont HL, Cooper KM, Laudadio C. Randomized, double-blind, placebo-controlled clinical trial of loperamide plus simethicone versus loperamide alone and simethicone alone in the treatment of acute diarrhea with gas-related abdominal discomfort. Curr Med Res Opin. 2007;23(5):1033–43.
23. Steffen R. Worldwide efficacy of bismuth subsalicylate in the treatment of traveler's diarrhea. Rev Infect Dis. 1990;12(Suppl 1):S80.
24. Lamberti LM, Walker CL, Chan KY, et al. Oral zinc supplementation for the treatment of acute diarrhea in children: a systematic review and meta-analysis. Nutrients. 2013;5(11):4715–40.

19 Hemorrhoids

Run Gan

19.1 Introduction

Hemorrhoids are a common cause of anal bleeding, itching, and pain. It is estimated that 4.4% of the population has symptomatic hemorrhoids, while the true prevalence of asymptomatic hemorrhoids is unknown [1]. Males and females are affected equally and peaks around age 45–65 years old. Hemorrhoids are uncommon before age 20.

Hemorrhoids result from dilation of the veins around the anus and rectum. Internal hemorrhoids originate above the dentate line [2]. They are covered by columnar epithelium, which lacks pain receptors. They are classified into four grades based on the degree of prolapse [3]:

- Grade I: No prolapse, just prominent blood vessels
- Grade II: Prolapse upon bearing down but spontaneous reduction
- Grade III: Prolapse upon bearing down requiring manual reduction
- Grade IV: Prolapse with inability to be manually reduced

External hemorrhoids occur below the dentate. They have somatic innervations and thus are sensitive to pain and temperature [3].

Risk factors for hemorrhoids include prolonged straining, constipation, diarrhea, pregnancy, and ascites.

R. Gan (✉)
Department of Community Health and Family Medicine, University of Florida College of Medicine, Gainesville, FL, USA
e-mail: rungan@ufl.edu

B. K. Desai et al. (eds.), *Primary Care for Emergency Physicians*,
https://doi.org/10.1007/978-3-031-64676-8_19

19.2 Differential

The differential diagnosis includes rectal cancer, condyloma, anal fissure, perianal abscess, IBD, and skin tags.

Hemorrhoidal bleeding is usually painless passage of bright red blood per rectum with a bowel movement. Painful defecation is usually not associated with hemorrhoids, unless it is thrombosed. Painful defecation is normally suggestive of an anorectal fissure, ulcer, abscess, rectal cancer, or anal polyp.

Systemic symptoms such as night sweats, fever, weight loss, and abdominal pain are not associated with hemorrhoids and are suggestive of an underlying malignancy, chronic infection, or inflammation. The presence of chronic diarrhea with hematochezia and tenesmus is suggestive of colitis. A change in the frequency, caliber, or consistency of stools is suggestive of a colorectal malignancy.

19.3 Physical Exam

Physical exam should include abdominal examination, inspection of the perineum, digital rectal examination, and anoscopy. Look for prolapsed internal hemorrhoids, condylomas, skin tags, neoplasms, and anal fissures. Digital rectal examination should be performed in the prone or left lateral position at rest and with straining. Anoscopy is usually required to look internally. On anoscopy, internal hemorrhoids appear as dilated purplish-blue veins, and prolapsed internal hemorrhoids appear as dark pink. External hemorrhoids appear less pink and, if thrombosed, are acutely tender with a purplish hue. Perianal skin tags are often remnants of previous external hemorrhoid. Some experts recommend colonoscopy for all patients older than 40 years who have hemorrhoidal symptoms and rectal bleeding. The American Society of Colon and Rectal Surgeons recommends taking the patient history and performing a physical examination with anoscopy and further endoscopic evaluation if there is concern for inflammatory bowel disease or cancer. A complete evaluation of the colon is warranted in the following groups [2]:

- Patients who are 50 years or older and have not had a complete examination of the colon within the past 10 years
- Patients who are 40 years or older and have not had a complete examination of the colon within the past 10 years and who have one first-degree relative in whom colorectal cancer or adenoma was diagnosed at age 60 years or younger.
- Patients who are 40 years or older and have not had a complete examination of the colon within the past 5 years and who have more than one first-degree relative in whom colorectal cancer or adenoma was diagnosed at age 60 years or younger
- Patients with iron deficiency anemia
- Patients who have a positive fecal occult blood test

19.4 Labs

Laboratory testing is not routinely recommended, but if it is performed and anemia or iron deficiency is identified, sigmoidoscopy or colonoscopy evaluation should be considered.

19.5 Treatment

Treatment of hemorrhoids usually begins with conservative therapy. This includes drinking more fluids and eating more fiber. Toilet habits such as prolong sitting and reading should be avoided. Analgesics taken orally or topically can be helpful. Low-dose hydrocortisone cream may improve itching and swelling. Sitz baths may improve anal hygiene, thus reducing irritation and pruritus.

If conservative therapy fails, next consider rubber band ligation, sclerotherapy, or surgery [4].

Rubber band ligation is typically recommended as the first-line treatment in those with grade 1–3 disease [5]. It is a procedure in which elastic bands are applied onto an internal hemorrhoid at least 1 cm above the dentate line to cut off its blood supply. Within 5–7 days, the withered hemorrhoid falls off. Cure rate has been found to be about 87% [1] with a complication rate of up to 3%.

Rubber band ligation is less effective than surgery in preventing recurrence of hemorrhoids, but it is associated with less pain and complications. Surgical options should be considered for thrombosed hemorrhoids or nonretractable prolapsed internal hemorrhoids.

Sclerotherapy involves the injection of a sclerosing agent, such as phenol, into the hemorrhoid. This causes the vein walls to collapse and the hemorrhoids to shrivel up. The success rate 4 years after treatment is about 70% [1].

Surgical excision remains a very effective approach for treatment of symptomatic hemorrhoids but is generally reserved for patients who failed an office-based procedure.

References

1. Rivadeneira DE, Steele SR, Ternent C, Chalasani S, Buie WD, Rafferty JL, Standards Practice Task Force of The American Society of Colon and Rectal, Surgeons. Practice parameters for the management of hemorrhoids (revised 2010). Dis Colon Rectum. 2011;54(9):1059–64. https://doi.org/10.1097/DCR.0b013e318225513d. PMID: 21825884.
2. Lawrence PF, Bell RM, Dayton MT, editors. Essentials of general surgery. 4th ed. Philadelphia: Williams & Wilkins; 2006. p. 329. isbn:9780781750035
3. Beck DE. The ASCRS textbook of colon and rectal surgery. 2nd ed. New York: Springer; 2011. p. 175. isbn:9781441915818.
4. Lorenzo-Rivero S. Hemorrhoids: diagnosis and current management. Am Surg. 2009;75(8):635–42. PMID: 19725283.

20 Acute Pelvic Pain

Morgan Killian

20.1 Introduction

Acute pelvic pain is commonly defined as pain in the pelvis or lower abdomen lasting less than 3 months [1]. Pelvic pain is a common complaint; over one-third of women of reproductive age will experience non-menstrual pelvic pain [2]. Because signs and symptoms are often nonspecific and insensitive, the workup and diagnosis of acute pelvic pain can be challenging. Also, the clinical presentation of each cause of pelvic pain may vary from patient to patient. Therefore, physicians should make an effort to keep a broad differential diagnosis when assessing patients with acute pelvic pain. It is critical to quickly identify emergent conditions of acute pelvic pain such as ectopic pregnancy, ovarian torsion, and appendiceal perforation. The consequences of missing these diagnoses are high and may result in infertility or death. Physicians must also consider both common causes of pelvic pain, such as urinary tract infections and cervicitis, and uncommon causes, such as heterotopic pregnancy and mesenteric adenitis.

20.2 Differential Diagnosis

The differential diagnosis of acute pelvic pain is vast and includes pathology from a wide variety of organ systems. The female pelvis includes many organs such as the vagina, uterus, fallopian tubes, ovaries, ureters, urinary bladder, sigmoid colon, rectum, and vascular, neurologic, and musculoskeletal structures. Any of these structures may be causing pelvic pain. Therefore, it is important to keep a broad differential. Age also impacts the probabilities of various etiologies. Categorizing conditions based on pregnancy status, organ systems, and the patient's age can be helpful.

M. Killian (✉)
University of Central Florida, Orlando, FL, USA

B. K. Desai et al. (eds.), *Primary Care for Emergency Physicians*,
https://doi.org/10.1007/978-3-031-64676-8_20

20.2.1 Gynecologic (Premenopausal)

- Cervix and uterus
  - Adenomyosis
  - Asherman's syndrome
  - Cervicitis
  - Dysmenorrhea
  - Endometriosis
  - Intrauterine device perforation
  - Leiomyoma (fibroid)
  - Post-procedure endometritis
  - Salpingitis
  - Uterine perforation
- Endocrine
  - Mittelschmerz
  - Primary dysmenorrhea
- Fallopian tube and ovary
  - Corpus luteum cyst
  - Ovarian torsion
  - Pelvic inflammatory disease
  - Round ligament mass
    - Lipoma
    - Teratoma
  - Ruptured ovarian cyst
  - Salpingitis
  - Tubo-ovarian abscess
- Vulva and vagina
  - Bartholin gland cyst/abscess
  - Contact vaginitis
  - Imperforate hymen
  - Transverse vaginal septum
  - Vaginismus
  - Vulvovaginitis
    - Bacterial vaginosis
    - Candida vaginitis
    - Trichomoniasis

20.2.2 Gynecologic (Postmenopausal)

- Atrophic vaginitis
- Malignancy
  - Endometrial
  - Ovarian
  - Uterine

- Uterine prolapse
- Uterine fibroids

20.2.3 Gastrointestinal

- Appendicitis
- Bowel obstruction
- Constipation
- Diverticulitis
- Intussusception
- Inflammatory bowel disease
- Inguinal hernia
- Irritable bowel syndrome
- Mesenteric adenitis
- Mesenteric ischemia
- Perirectal abscess
- Volvulus

20.2.4 Genitourinary

- Cystitis
- Interstitial cystitis
- Pyelonephritis
- Urethral diverticulum
- Urinary retention
- Urolithiasis

20.2.5 Musculoskeletal

- Muscular strain or sprain
- Pelvic fracture

20.2.6 Obstetric

- Abortion
  - Threatened
  - Inevitable
  - Incomplete
  - Complete
  - Missed
  - Septic

- Braxton Hicks contractions
- Corpus luteum hematoma
- Fertility treatment-related
  - Heterotopic pregnancy
  - Ovarian hyperstimulation syndrome
- Incarcerated gravid uterus
- Normal labor
- Ovarian vein thrombosis
- Preterm labor
- Placental abruption
- Postpartum endometritis
- Pubic symphysis separation
- Round ligament stretch
- Ruptured ectopic pregnancy
- Uterine abruption
- Wound infections (Caesarian section, lacerations, or episiotomies)

20.2.7 Others

- Domestic violence
- Lead poisoning
- Porphyria
- Sexual abuse

20.2.8 Psychiatric

- Depression
- Drug-seeking
- Malingering
- Somatization disorders

20.2.9 Vascular

- Abdominal aortic aneurysm
- Aortic dissection
- Ovarian vein thrombosis
- Sickle cell crisis
- Septic pelvic thrombophlebitis

20.3 History

A thorough history and physical examination is essential to the diagnosis of acute pelvic pain. Eliciting specific information about the patient's clinical situation and correlating that information with the patient's physical examination allow a physician to choose the appropriate laboratory testing and imaging modalities in order to identify the cause of that patient's pain.

Important historical features to elicit include:

- Location of pain
  - Where is the pain located?
    - Right-sided pelvic pain can be suggestive of conditions such as appendicitis.
    - Left-sided pelvic pain can be suggestive of conditions such as diverticulitis.
      - Beware that some conditions can present as either right- or left-sided pelvic pain, such as ovarian torsion, tubo-ovarian abscess, or ectopic pregnancy.
    - Suprapubic pain can be suggestive of conditions such as cystitis.
- Radiation of pain
  - Where does the pain radiate?
    - Pain that radiates to the groin can be suggestive of urolithiasis or ovarian torsion.
    - Pain that radiates to the back can be suggestive of aortic dissection.
    - Many conditions have pain that does not radiate.
- Quality of pain
  - What does the pain feel like? (Pressure, sharp, crampy, burning, colicky, etc.)
    - Burning pain can be suggestive of cystitis.
    - Colicky pain can be suggestive of urolithiasis.
- Onset of pain
  - How long has the patient had the pain?
  - What was the patient doing when the pain first began?
  - Was the pain gradual or sudden in onset?
  - Since the pain began, has it gotten better, worse, or stayed the same?
- Timing/frequency of pain
  - When does the pain occur?
    - Pain that occurs during the middle of each menstrual cycle can be suggestive of Mittelschmerz.
  - How often does the pain occur?
    - Colicky pain that waxes and wanes can be suggestive of urolithiasis.
- Associated symptoms
  - A thorough review of systems allows a physician to identify associated symptoms in order to narrow the differential diagnosis. For example:
    - Right lower quadrant abdominal pain that is associated with a history of multiple sex partners, history of sexually transmitted diseases, and vaginal discharge is suspicious for tubo-ovarian abscess.

Right lower quadrant abdominal pain that is associated with anorexia, nausea, and vomiting is more suggestive of appendicitis.

- Previous episodes
  - If a patient has had previous symptoms similar to this present episode, it may change your differential diagnosis.
  - It is important to keep the differential open in order not to miss other diagnoses that can present similarly. For example, an abdominal aortic aneurysm or dissection may present similar to a kidney stone.
- Aggravating factors
  - What makes the pain worse? (Eating, position, activity, intercourse, urinating, etc.)
- Relieving factors
  - What makes the pain better? (Positions, holding pressure, medications, etc.)
- Gynecologic history
  - Last menstrual period

    Patients who have missed menstrual cycles may be pregnant. This also expands the differential diagnosis to include ectopic pregnancy, miscarriage, and more.
  - Menstrual cycle and deviations from normal menstrual cycle

    Age of menarche?

    Cycle length?

    Amount of vaginal bleeding?

    Pain with menses?

    Age of menopause? (If applicable)

      Vaginal bleeding in postmenopausal women can be suggestive of endometrial cancer.
  - Contraception use

    Type of contraception? (Oral, IUD, barrier, rhythm method, none)
  - Sexual history

    Sexually active? If yes, with men or women or both?

    Recent new sexual partners?

    History of sexually transmitted infections?

      A history of sexually transmitted infections can increase the likelihood of developing an ectopic pregnancy [3].

      Pelvic inflammatory disease is generally thought to be a complication of sexually transmitted infections, but cases have been reported of virgin women being diagnosed with PID [4]. Therefore, pelvic inflammatory disease should still be considered as a possible cause of pelvic pain in all women regardless of sexual history.
  - Cervical cancer screening

    HPV vaccination?

    Previous pap smears?

      History of abnormal pap smears? If yes, what diagnostic procedures were performed?

    History of cervical cancer?

  - Pregnancies and outcomes
    - History of pregnancies? If yes, how many?
    - Results of pregnancies? (Miscarriage, termination, preterm, term, full-term, natural birth, Caesarian)
    - Complications during pregnancy or delivery?
    - History of fertility-enhancing medications?
- Past medical history
  - A thorough past medical history is an important component of the history. A patient's past medical history can place a patient at risk for certain conditions that cause pelvic pain.
- Past surgical history
  - Previous surgeries can increase the likelihood of certain diagnoses. For example:
    - History of abdominal surgeries, even laparoscopic surgeries, increases the risk of bowel obstruction [5].
    - History of pelvic organ surgery increases the risk for ectopic pregnancy [6].
    - IUD insertion is associated with a sixfold increase in the risk of developing pelvic inflammatory disease for the next 20 days [7].

20.4 Physical Examination

The physical examination should include vital signs, abdominal examination, and pelvic examination.

Vital signs should be assessed as soon as possible. Fever can be suggestive of infectious etiologies. Hypotension and tachycardia in the setting of pelvic pain should raise concern for surgical emergencies such as ruptured ectopic pregnancy.

The abdominal examination is important in the diagnosis of acute pelvic pain. Abdominal rigidity, rebound, and guarding can be indicative of a surgical abdomen and may warrant prompt consultation.

A pelvic examination must also be performed in the setting of pelvic pain, even though it may be uncomfortable in a patient experiencing pelvic pain. One of the only exceptions is in pregnant patients greater than 20 weeks' gestation. These patients should have a transabdominal ultrasound prior to pelvic exam in order to ensure the location of the placenta. The pelvic exam should consist of both a speculum and a bimanual examination. The examination begins with inspection of the external genitalia for discoloration, rashes, swelling, or lesions. The physician should inspect the urethra, Skene's glands, and Bartholin glands for abnormalities. Next, a speculum is inserted to examine the vaginal walls for erythema, blood, lacerations, discharge, swelling, or foreign body. The blades of the speculum are then opened to evaluate the cervix for erythema, blood, ulcerations, and masses and to assess the os (open vs closed). The speculum is then removed, and a bimanual examination is performed to assess the cervix for motion tenderness, the uterus for size, position, and tenderness; and the adnexa for masses or tenderness.

Although it is an integral component in the evaluation of acute pelvic pain, the pelvic exam does have several limitations. Physical examination findings tend to not be specific for only one etiology. For example, cervical motion tenderness has been shown to be nonspecific for pelvic inflammatory disease. Cervical motion tenderness has been found to be present in 25% of cases of appendicitis and 50% of cases of ectopic pregnancies [8]. Additionally, the absence of physical examination findings should not exclude certain diagnoses. For example, one study demonstrated that the detection of adnexal mass in women with a known adnexal mass has been shown to have sensitivities as low as 16–28% [9]. Examination findings also vary from provider to provider. A recent study using emergency medicine physicians showed that there was only agreement of positive findings during pelvic examination in 17–33% of examinations [10].

20.5 Laboratory Testing

The history and physical exam should guide the laboratory testing. Nevertheless, all women of reproductive age should receive a beta-subunit of human chorionic gonadotropin (B-hCG) to assess for pregnancy. Other commonly ordered tests include complete blood count (CBC) with differential to assess for infectious etiologies and to establish a baseline hemoglobin and hematocrit, urinalysis with culture to assess for pyuria and hematuria, and nucleic amplification tests to assess for chlamydial and gonorrheal infections. Cervical swabs and urine samples for nucleic amplification of chlamydia and gonorrhea have been shown to have similar sensitivities and specificities for detection of chlamydia and gonorrhea [11].

20.6 Imaging

The differential diagnoses should also guide the physician's imaging choice. Physician should select imaging modalities that offer the greatest diagnostic value and the least amount of radiation exposure. Although computed tomography (CT) is more sensitive than ultrasound in assessing acute pelvic pain, ultrasound examination is the preferred initial imaging modality for most patients with acute pelvic pain given its low cost, absence of radiation exposure, and high sensitivity. One study demonstrated that using ultrasonography first, with CT only used when ultrasound results were negative or inconclusive, provided the best diagnostic value while subjecting the patient to the lowest amount of radiation possible [12]. However, physicians should choose a MRI in pregnant patients with a nondiagnostic ultrasound.

Ultrasonography with Doppler venous flow is the imaging modality of choice when evaluating for ovarian torsion. Absent venous flow to the ovary on ultrasound is 99.6% specific for ovarian torsion. However, due to the possibility of partial or intermittent torsion, venous flow to the ovary on ultrasound is only 72.1% sensitive for excluding ovarian torsion. Flow to the ovary can be present even when torsion is present due to the dual blood supply of the ovary. Therefore, ovarian torsion cannot be reliably excluded by ultrasound if suspicion is high despite a normal ultrasound [13].

Physicians must exclude ectopic pregnancy in all pregnant patients presenting with pelvic pain. When the serum B-hCG is above the discriminatory zone of 1500 IU/L, a transvaginal ultrasound should confirm an intrauterine pregnancy. If an ultrasound cannot confirm an intrauterine pregnancy, physicians should suspect an ectopic pregnancy. One meta-analysis determined that an empty uterus on ultrasound is associated with a sensitivity of 81.1% and a specificity of 79.5% for ectopic pregnancy. Similarly, the sensitivities and specificities of the presence of a pseudosac are 5.5% and 94.2%, the presence of adnexal mass are 63.5% and 91.4%, and the presence of free fluid 47.2% and 92.3%, respectively, for ectopic pregnancy. Therefore, ultrasound has strong specificity for diagnosing ectopic pregnancy but poorer sensitivity for excluding ectopic pregnancy [14].

20.7 Treatment

The treatment of acute pelvic pain varies with respect to its etiology.

Life-threatening etiologies such as ectopic pregnancy, placental abruption, and hemorrhagic ovarian cyst should be treated emergently with fluid, blood products, and possibly surgical intervention. On the other hand, women with acute pelvic pain and normal physical examination, laboratory studies, and imaging will improve without any intervention and can be safely discharged with primary care and/or obstetrician/gynecologist follow-up. Such disease etiologies include pelvic adhesions, endometriosis, and subclinical pelvic inflammatory disease [15].

20.7.1 Surgical Intervention

Surgical intervention, such as laparoscopy or laparotomy, is the treatment of choice for most emergent causes of acute pelvic pain. Laparoscopy is usually preferred over laparotomy due to shorter hospital stays, less postoperative pain, and faster recovery. In many cases, laparoscopy is both therapeutic and diagnostic, such as in the setting of a nondiagnostic transvaginal ultrasound with concern for ectopic pregnancy. Laparoscopy is the definitive treatment for the removal of ectopic pregnancies, detorsion of ovarian torsion, and washout for ruptured tubo-ovarian abscess [16]. However, laparotomy is preferred in hemodynamically unstable patients.

20.7.2 Ovarian Cysts

Ruptured ovarian cysts are managed according to whether they are uncomplicated or complicated. Complicated ovarian cyst rupture occurs when there is hemodynamic instability, evidence of infection, or suspicion of malignancy; this is managed with laparoscopy. Uncomplicated ovarian cyst rupture occurs when there is no hemodynamic instability, evidence of infection, or suspicion of malignancy. It is managed conservatively with observation and pain control including NSAIDs.

20.7.3 Infections

Infectious etiologies should be treated with antibiotics. The Centers for Disease Control and Prevention recommends empiric treatment of pelvic inflammatory disease with antibiotics that are effective against *N. gonorrhoeae* and *C. trachomatis* in women who are at increased risk of sexually transmitted infections or for whom clinical suspicion is high for pelvic inflammatory disease. This is typically treated with one 500 mg intramuscular dose of ceftriaxone, with recommendation for co-treatment of chlamydia with 100 mg doxycycline twice a day for 7 days [17]. Vulvovaginal candidiasis is typically treated with topical antifungals such as clotrimazole and miconazole (one applicator nightly intravaginally for 7 nights) or with oral antifungals such as fluconazole (single dose of 150 mg). Bacterial vaginosis is typically treated with oral metronidazole (750 mg twice daily for 7 days) [18] or topical clindamycin cream (one applicator nightly for 3–7 nights). Trichomoniasis is typically treated with oral metronidazole (single dose of 2 g, two doses of 1 g, or 250 mg three times a day for 7 days) [18]. Uncomplicated cystitis can be treated with several different medications including nitrofurantoin, trimethoprim/sulfamethoxazole, or fluoroquinolones.

20.7.4 Endometriosis

Endometriosis can be a cause of debilitating pelvic pain. Management consists of controlling the patient's pain and preventing flares. Mild to moderate pain can be treated with NSAIDs and estrogen-progesterone oral contraceptive pills. Severe symptoms that do not respond to these therapies can be treated with ovarian suppression via GnRH analogs. If a patient still experiences pain secondary to endometriosis, the definitive treatment is obliteration of the extrauterine endometrial tissue by laparoscopy [19].

References

1. Kruszka PS, Kruszka SJ. Evaluation of acute pelvic pain in women. Am Fam Physician. 2010;82(2):141–7.
2. Walls RM, Hockberger RS, Gausche-Hill M. Rosen's emergency medicine concepts and clinical practice. Elsevier; 2018.
3. Moore MS, Golden MR. Assessing trends in chlamydia positivity and gonorrhea incidence and their associations with the incidence of pelvic inflammatory disease and ectopic pregnancy in Washington state, 1988-2010. Sex Transm Dis. 2016;43(1):2–8.
4. Cho HW, Koo YJ, Min KJ, Hong JH, Lee JK. Pelvic inflammatory disease in virgin women with tubo-ovarian abscess: a single-center experience and literature review [published online

ahead of print August 7, 2015]. J Pediatr Adolesc Gynecol. http://www.sciencedirect.com/science/article/pii/S1083318815002922. Accessed 31 Jan 2016.

5. Jafari MD, Jafari F, et al. Adhesive small bowel obstruction in the United States: has laparoscopy made an impact? Am Surg. 2015;81(10):1028–33.
6. Barnhart KT, Sammel MD, Garcia CR, et al. Risk factors for ectopic pregnancy in women with symptomatic first-trimester pregnancies. Fertil Steril. 2006;86(1):36–43.
7. Farley TM, Rosenberg MJ, Rowe PJ, Chen JH, Meirik O. Intrauterine devices and pelvic inflammatory disease: an international perspective. Lancet. 1992;339(8796):785–8.
8. Quan M. Diagnosis of acute pelvic pain. J Fam Pract. 1992;35(4):422–32.
9. Padilla LA, Radosevich DM, Milad MP. Accuracy of the pelvic examination in detecting adnexal masses. Obstet Gynecol. 2000;96(4):593–8.
10. Close RJ, Sachs CJ, Dyne PL. Reliability of bimanual pelvic examinations performed in emergency departments. West J Med. 2001;175(4):240–5.
11. Lunny C, Taylor D, et al. Self-collected versus clinician-collected sampling for chlamydia and gonorrhea screening: a systematic review and meta-analysis. PLoS One. 2015;10(7):e0132776.
12. Laméris W, van Randen A, van Es HW, et al.; OPTIMA Study Group. Imaging strategies for detection of urgent conditions in patients with acute abdominal pain: diagnostic accuracy study. BMJ. 2009;338:b2431.
13. Rostamzadeh A, Mirfendereski S, et al. Diagnostic efficacy of sonography for diagnosis of ovarian torsion. Pak J Med Sci. 2014;30(2):413–6.
14. Richardson A, Gallos I, et al. Accuracy of first-trimester ultrasound in diagnosis of tubal ectopic pregnancy in the absence of an obvious extrauterine embryo: systematic review and meta-analysis. Ultrasound Obstet Gynecol. 2016;47(1):28–37.
15. Harris RD, et al. Clinical outcome in female patients with pelvic pain and normal pelvic US findings. Radiology. 2000;216:440.
16. Promecene PA. Laparoscopy in gynecologic emergencies. Semin Laparosc Surg. 2002;9(1):64–75.
17. Centers for Disease Control and Prevention. Update to CDC's treatment guidelines for gonococcal infection, 2020. 2020. cdc.gov/mmwr/volumes/69/wr/mm6950a6.htm.
18. Mayo Clinic. Metronidazole (oral route). 2022. https://www.mayoclinic.org/drugs-supplements/metronidazole-oral-route/proper-use/drg-20064745.
19. Practice Committee of the American Society for Reproductive Medicine. Treatment of pelvic pain associated with endometriosis: a committee opinion. Fertil Steril. 2014;101(4):927–35.

Dysmenorrhea

21

Emily Weeks

21.1 Introduction

Dysmenorrhea is defined as painful menstruation occurring just before or during menses. It is the most common gynecologic condition among women of reproductive age [1]. In surveys, 50–90% of reproductive-aged women worldwide describe experiencing painful menstrual periods [2]. Despite high prevalence of disease, many patients do not seek professional treatment. For clinical purposes, dysmenorrhea is further divided into primary and secondary dysmenorrhea (Fig. 21.1). Primary dysmenorrhea refers to the presence of recurrent lower abdominal cramps/pain that occurs during menses in the absence of pelvic pathology and normally occurs within the first 24 months of menarche [3]. The most widely accepted explanation for the pathogenesis of primary dysmenorrhea is the overproduction of uterine prostaglandins (PG). Secondary dysmenorrhea has the same presenting features but occurs in the setting of identifiable or underlying pelvic pathology as the suspected origin of symptoms, such as endometriosis, adenomyosis, pelvic inflammatory disease, or uterine fibroids [3]. Secondary dysmenorrhea often has additional associated clinical features that distinguish it from primary dysmenorrhea, such as dyspareunia. Dysmenorrhea is responsible for considerable economic losses due to the costs of medication, medical care, and decreased productivity [4].

21.2 Risk Factors for Dysmenorrhea

- Primary Dysmenorrhea
  - Age < 30 years
  - Body mass index <20 kg/m^2

E. Weeks (✉)
University of Central Florida, Orlando, FL, USA
e-mail: emily.weeksgraham@envisionhealth.com

B. K. Desai et al. (eds.), *Primary Care for Emergency Physicians*,
https://doi.org/10.1007/978-3-031-64676-8_21

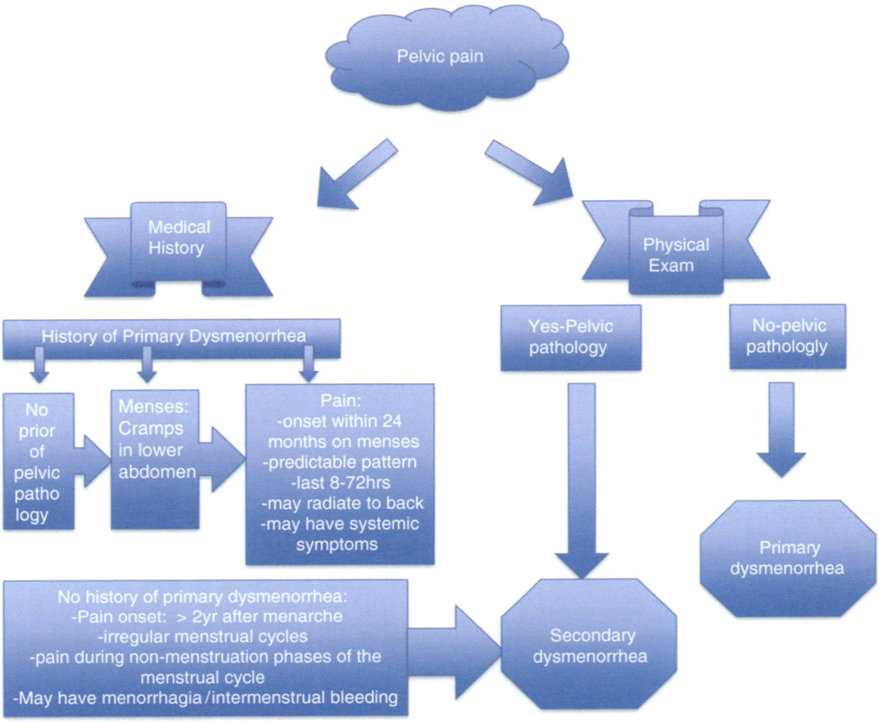

Fig. 21.1 Primary vs. secondary dysmenorrhea flow diagram

  - Smoking
  - Menarche before age 12
  - Longer menstrual cycles/duration of bleeding and irregular or heavy menstrual flow
  - History of sex assault [2]
  - Younger age at first childbirth and higher parity associated with a reduced risk
- Secondary Dysmenorrhea
  - Onset of pain after age 25–30 and/or after years of normal cycles
  - Pain during menses that does not resolve after the first few days
  - Pain at times other than menses
  - Dyspareunia
  - Dyschezia
  - Progressively worsening symptoms [5]

Dysmenorrhea is positively associated with stress related to both work and general life, as well as with family history of dysmenorrhea [6].

Dysmenorrhea is inversely related to age, parity or number of live births, and oral contraception use [6].

21.3 Differential Diagnosis

- Mittelschmerz
- Endometriosis
- Adenomyosis
- Cervical stenosis
- Gastroenterology causes
- Urinary tract infection
- Interstitial cystitis
- Pelvic congestive syndrome
- Leiomyoma
- Musculoskeletal causes
- Intrauterine device (IUD)
- Mullerian malformations
- Psychogenic disorders
- Miscarriage
- Ovarian cyst
- Ovarian torsion

21.4 Common Complaints and Red Flags

- Pain typically lasts 8–72 h [3].
- Pain is most severe during the first or second day of menses [5].
- Systemic symptoms: nausea, vomiting, diarrhea, fatigue, and insomnia [5].
- Patients with irritable bowel syndrome (IBS) more likely to experience dysmenorrhea [7].
- High rates of absenteeism from school/work, fatigue, and sleepiness may stem from inadequately treated dysmenorrhea.
- Red flags:
  - Pain lasting more than 72 h
  - Acute abdomen
  - Abnormal vital signs
  - Fever
  - Positive pregnancy test
  - Palpable abdominal or pelvic mass
  - Severe anemia

21.5 History

When evaluating dysmenorrhea, it is important to differentiate primary dysmenorrhea from secondary dysmenorrhea, as secondary causes often require further evaluation and treatment of the underlying pathology. Severe pain sufficient to limit daily activities is less common, affecting approximately 7–15% of women [6].

Menstrual pain is referred to the abdomen in 70–90% of patients and to the lower back in 40% of patients [3].

Important historical features to elicit include:

- History of sexually transmitted infection
- Pregnancies
- Pelvic pathology
- Tobacco or alcohol use
- Sedentary lifestyle
- Family history of pelvic pain
- Dietary habits
- Menstrual history:
  - Age at menarche and at onset of menstrual pain
  - Menstrual cycles: frequency, duration, and amount (heavy/moderate/light)
  - Regularity
  - Timing between onset of symptoms and menses
  - Severity and location of pain
  - Associated symptoms
  - Impact of symptoms on daily activities
  - Previous medication use (dose, duration, efficacy)

21.6 Physical Examination

- Vital sign assessment (rule out)
  - Febrile
  - Hypotension
  - Tachycardia
- Abdominal exam (rule out)
  - Guarding/rebound tenderness
  - Abdominal mass
- Pelvic exam—if sexually active, severe symptoms (grade 3) or symptoms suggestive of pelvic pathology (rule out)
  - Cervix—mucopurulent discharge, friability, and cervical motion tenderness
  - Uterus—asymmetrical, enlarged, and exquisitely tender
  - Adnexa—fullness or passes and exquisitely tender
  - Products of conception in vagina or protruding from cervix
  - Vaginal wet mount/Pap smear when appropriate
- Urine HCG
- Urinalysis

While lab tests, imaging studies, and laparoscopy are not mandatory to exclude secondary dysmenorrhea, they may be considered if underlying pelvic pathology is suspected.

21.7 Introduction to Treatment

Increased levels of circulating PGF2α and PGE_2 lead to increased myometrial contraction, vasoconstriction, and hypersensitization of pain fibers [3]. On account of the PG-based etiology of primary dysmenorrhea, the present most common pharmacologic treatment for dysmenorrhea is nonsteroidal anti-inflammatory drugs (NSAIDS) [8].

21.8 Pharmacologic Treatment

21.8.1 NSAIDS: First-Line Therapy

Various formulations of NSAIDS have comparable efficacy for dysmenorrhea, and pain relief is successfully achieved in 64–100% of women [3].

Nonsteroidal anti-inflammatory drugs (NSAIDS)
Naproxen
Ibuprofen
Mefenamic acid
Diclofenac

Pitfalls

1. May increase risk of cardiovascular thrombotic events
2. May increase risk of stroke
3. May increase risk of gastric ulcer/bleed and intestinal perforation
4. Caution in asthma
5. Caution in dehydration

21.8.2 Hormonal Contraceptives: Second-Line Therapy

Suppress ovulation and reduce thickness of the endometrial lining of the uterus, thereby reducing the volume of menstrual fluid [8]. This form of therapy includes hormonal intrauterine devices (IUD) [3].

Pitfalls

1. Increased risk of thrombotic event
2. Increased risk of cardiovascular side effects with cigarette smoking
3. Contraindicated with known thrombophilia
4. Contraindicated if migraine headaches with aura*
5. Contraindicated in estrogen- or progestin-dependent cancers

6. Caution in hepatic disease

**IUDs are not contraindicated with migraine headaches with aura but should be used with caution.*

21.9 Nonpharmacologic Treatment

21.9.1 Abdominal Heat Wrap: First-Line Therapy

Found to be as effective as ibuprofen and more effective than acetaminophen in relieving dysmenorrhea pain [9]. Can decrease time to pain relief when used in combination with NSAIDs [5].

21.9.2 Exercise [5]

Pitfalls

1. Thermal skin damage when heat wraps used inappropriately.
2. Exercise-induced injuries may occur.

21.10 Alternative Medicine/Treatments [5]

*Transcutaneous electrical nervous stimulation**
*Acupuncture/acupressure**
*Low-fat diet**
*Chinese herb preparations**
**Limited evidence to support*

Pitfalls

1. Expensive
2. Controversial

References

1. Coco AS. Primary dysmenorrhea. Am Fam Physician. 1999;60(2):489–96.
2. Andersch B, Milsom I. An epidemiologic study of young women with dysmenorrhea. Am J Obstet Gynecol. 1982;144(6):655–60. https://doi.org/10.1016/0002-9378(82)90433-1.
3. Lacovides S, Avidon I, Baker FC. What we know about primary dysmenorrhea today: a critical review. Hum Reprod Update. 2015;21(6):762–78. https://doi.org/10.1093/humupd/dmv039.
4. Lobo RA, Gershenson DM, Lentz GM, Valea FA. Comprehensive gynecology. Elsevier; 2017.
5. Roberts SC, Hodgkiss C, DiBenedetto A, Lee E. Managing dysmenorrhea in young women. Nurse Pract. 2012;37(7):47–52. https://doi.org/10.1097/01.npr.0000415245.88638.bf.

6. Ju H, Jones M, Mishra G. The prevalence and risk factors of dysmenorrhea. Epidemiol Rev. 2014;36:104–13. https://doi.org/10.1093/epirev/mxt009.
7. Olafsdottir LB, Gudjonsson H, Jonsdottir HH, Björnsson E, Thjodleifsson B. Natural history of irritable bowel syndrome in women and dysmenorrhea: a 10-year follow-up study. Gastroenterol Res Pract. 2012;2012:534204. https://doi.org/10.1155/2012/534204.
8. Ruoff G, Lema M. Strategies in pain management: new and potential indications for COX-2 specific inhibitors. J Pain Symptom Manag. 2003;25(2 Suppl):S21–31. https://doi.org/10.1016/s0885-3924(02)00628-0.
9. Akin MD, Weingand KW, Hengehold DA, Goodale MB, Hinkle RT, Smith RP. Continuous low-level topical heat in the treatment of dysmenorrhea. Obstet Gynecol. 2001;97(3):343–9. https://doi.org/10.1016/s0029-7844(00)01163-7.

Back Pain

22

Shane Dluzneski and Josh Walker

22.1 Introduction

Worldwide, back pain is one of the most frequent disorders people experience, with low back pain specifically accounting for the majority of complaints. In fact, the Global Burden of Disease study ranked low back pain as the number one cause of years lived with disability [1]. In the USA, back pain has a lifetime prevalence of close to 80%, and spinal disorders are in the top five most common primary diagnoses for office visits [2].

For the emergency physician, acute back pain is of particular importance, although chronic back pain with an acute flare can precipitate an emergency department (ED) visit as well. While low back pain typically originates from the lumbosacral spinous structures and para-spinous musculature, thoracic back pain can often represent referred pain from the viscera and should warrant careful consideration.

Because back pain is so frequently encountered in both the primary care and ER settings, it poses a substantial financial burden on the healthcare system [3] and is a common source for unnecessary testing, referrals, and inappropriate prescribing practices. Therefore, differentiating back pain that is likely to spontaneously resolve versus that which may represent a more ominous underlying pathology is an important skill for patient care as well as for appropriate resource utilization.

22.2 Risk Factors for Low Back Pain [4]

- Obesity
- Physical inactivity

S. Dluzneski · J. Walker (✉)
University of Central Florida, Orlando, FL, USA
e-mail: joshua.walker@envisionhealth.com

B. K. Desai et al. (eds.), *Primary Care for Emergency Physicians*,
https://doi.org/10.1007/978-3-031-64676-8_22

- Age >30
- Work that requires heavy lifting, twisting, bending, or whole body vibration (e.g., truck driving)
- Arthritis
- Osteoporosis
- Pregnancy
- Stress or depression
- Bad posture
- Smoking

22.3 History and Differential Diagnosis

When obtaining history for low back pain with or without sciatica, it is particularly important to ask about red flag symptoms. The presence of red flag symptoms indicates the potential for a more complicated underlying pathology affecting the spine which will likely require additional workup with diagnostic imaging and lab tests. The following list represents historical items that are suggestive of a more serious underlying condition [5]:

- Infection—0.1% of cases
  - Immunosuppression
  - Intravenous drug use
  - Prolonged corticosteroid use
  - Urinary infection
  - Fever
  - Pain not improved with rest or 6 weeks of conservative measures
  - Unrelenting night pain
- Cancer—0.7% of cases
  - Prior history of cancer or present cancer diagnosis
  - Unexplained weight loss
  - Pain not improved with rest or 6 weeks of conservative measures
  - Unrelenting night pain
- Spinal fracture (including osteoporotic compression fractures)—4% of cases
  - History of significant trauma
  - Prolonged corticosteroid use
  - History of osteoporosis especially in the setting of a fall or heavy lift
  - Elderly age group especially in the setting of a fall or heavy lift
- Cauda equina syndrome or severe neurologic compromise
  - Acute urinary retention or overflow incontinence
  - Loss of anal sphincter tone or fecal incontinence
  - Progressive motor weakness of lower extremities
  - Saddle anesthesia

- Inflammatory back pain (ankylosing spondylitis, reactive arthritis, psoriatic arthritis)—0.3% of cases
  - Progressive worsening of pain beyond 3 months.
  - Age less than 40.
  - Predominant morning stiffness.
  - Pain improves with activity.
  - Associated rash.
  - Other joint pains (especially of hands and feet).
  - Antecedent flu-like illness, STI, or gastrointestinal illness.
  - Eye complaints (painful, red eyes).

Although the above conditions are important to address in the history, almost 90% of low back complaints are related to mechanical problems originating from damage to the musculo-ligamentous structures or intervertebral disks [5]:

- Lumbar strain or sprain—≥70% of cases
  - Diffuse, nonspecific pain of lumbar muscles
  - Radiation to buttocks
  - Worsened with activity
  - Improvement with rest and/or OTC pain relievers
- Degenerative disk or facet disease—10% of cases
  - History of chronic back pain
  - Pain localized closer to lumbar spine but still nonspecific
  - Worsened with activity
  - Improvement with rest and/or OTC pain relievers
  - Age >50
  - Herniated disk—4% of cases
  - Radicular pain (often radiates below the knee, but the specific pattern depends on the affected vertebral level).
  - Leg pain often exceeds back pain.
  - Age 20–50.
  - Unilateral leg weakness (especially activities involving dorsi-/plantar flexion).
- Spinal stenosis—3% of cases
  - Aching in thighs or calves with walking (i.e., "neurogenic claudication").
  - Pain is bilateral.
  - Exacerbated by spine extension (e.g., walking downhill or lying flat).
  - Alleviated by spine flexion (e.g., walking uphill or leaning on shopping cart).
  - Pain improved with sitting.
- Spondylolisthesis
  - Worsened with activity
  - Improvement with rest
  - Can present similarly to degenerative disk disease or spinal stenosis
  - Usually discovered on imaging

Non-spinal and visceral disorders account for about 2% of cases of back pain (although rarely as isolated back pain) [5], so although they are a relatively uncommon cause of back pain, they are important to recognize because they often require specific treatment:

- Prostatitis
  - Dysuria
  - Fever
  - Pain with sitting
  - Lower abdominal/pelvic pain
- Pelvic inflammatory disease
  - Vaginal discharge
  - Fever
  - History of STIs or multiple sex partners
  - Lower abdominal/pelvic pain
- Cystitis
  - Dysuria
  - Urinary frequency
  - Fever
- Endometriosis
  - Dyspareunia
  - Pain worse at time of menses
  - Lower abdominal/pelvic pain
- Pyelonephritis
  - Localized to unilateral flank/thoracic back
  - Fever
  - Nausea and/or vomiting
- Nephrolithiasis
  - Localized to unilateral flank/thoracic back
  - Nausea and/or vomiting
  - Hematuria
  - Radiation to ipsilateral inguinal region
- Aortic aneurysm
  - Epigastric pain
  - Age >65
  - History of smoking
- Aortic dissection
  - Ripping/tearing quality to pain
  - History of HTN
  - Anterior chest pain
- Pancreatitis
  - Pain worse with eating.
  - Pain radiates from epigastrium.
  - History of alcohol abuse, gallstones, or severe hypertriglyceridemia.
  - Localized to mid-back.

  - Nausea and/or vomiting.
- Peptic ulcer
  - Heavy NSAID use.
  - Pain worse with eating.
  - Melena.
  - Pain radiates from epigastrium.
  - Nausea and/or vomiting.
- Cholecystitis
  - Pain radiates to right scapula.
  - Pain radiates from abdominal RUQ.
  - Nausea and/or vomiting.
- Shingles
  - Localized to unilateral flank/thoracic back in specific dermatome
  - Usually associated with blistering rash but pain can precede rash

While low back pain accounts for the majority of back pain syndromes, thoracic back pain is by no means rare. Fortunately, with few exceptions, low back pain and thoracic back pain share the same etiologies and therefore also share historical features that help formulate a differential. It should be noted that degenerative processes which commonly lead to lumbar pain are much less likely to occur in the thoracic spine, as opposed to fractures (especially compression fractures) which are relatively more common in the thoracic spine [6].

A final important aspect of the history for back pain is the possibility of opioid addiction. Some patients may be presenting with complaints of back pain as a way to receive narcotic pain medications either for personal abuse or for resale illegally. Some prototypical warning signs of drug-seeking behavior are as follows [7]:

- Multiple visits for the same complaint
- Inability to focus on anything other than the medicine
- Lost/stolen prescription
- "Doctor unavailable"
- No PCP contact
- "Allergic" to narcotic alternatives
  - NSAIDs
  - Muscle relaxants
  - Neuropathic agents
- Requests specific narcotics
- "Unbearable" pain
- Overly creative requests
- Upset when asked clarifying questions about pain
  - Location
  - Duration
  - Onset
- Night or weekend presentation

22.4 Physical Exam

For the emergency physician, the physical exam should focus on evaluating those conditions that may require urgent surgical consultation or systemic therapy (i.e., antibiotics):

- Vital sign assessment
  - Fever or hypothermia may suggest osteomyelitis, diskitis, or spinal abscess.
  - Tachycardia and/or hypertension may correspond to the degree of pain.
    - Response may be muted if on beta-blocker therapy.
    - Patients in opiate withdrawal may present this way also.
- MSK and neurological exam [8]
  - Straight leg raise
    - Radicular pain in affected leg being raised at 60° or less suggests disk herniation.
  - Crossed straight leg raise
    - Radicular pain in affected leg while contralateral (i.e., non-affected) leg is raised suggests disk herniation.
  - Range of movement
    - Reduced flexion of spine suggests ankylosing spondylitis.
    - Pain with prolonged extension of spine (30 s) suggests spinal stenosis.
  - Palpation of spine
    - Point tenderness over spine suggests fracture, malignancy, or infection.
  - Strength testing
    - Weakness in great toe, ankle, or quadriceps suggests disk herniation.
    - Diminished anal sphincter tone can be seen with cauda equina syndrome.
  - Reflexes
    - Hyporeflexia at Achilles or patellar tendons suggests nerve root involvement such as with disk herniation or spinal stenosis.
    - Hyperreflexia suggests spinal cord involvement such as with metastatic disease, infection, or fracture.
    - Positive Babinski test, lower extremity spasticity, or presence of clonus indicates possible spinal cord involvement.
  - Sensation
    - Diminished sensation especially along a dermatome suggests nerve root impingement.
  - Gait assessment
    - Inability to heel walk suggests L5 nerve involvement.
    - Inability to toe walk suggests S1 nerve involvement.
- Skin exam
  - Blistering rash in dermatomal distribution suggests shingles.
- Abdominal exam

   - Palpation
     Tenderness in epigastrium or RUQ may suggest pancreatitis or cholecystitis, respectively.
     Large pulsatile mass in periumbilical area suggests abdominal aortic aneurysm.
- Psychiatric evaluation
   - Assess for depression and/or anxiety.
     May indicate somatization of back pain

22.5 Diagnostic Workup

In general, acute low back pain and/or radiculopathy that does not present with red flag features (see section entitled "History and Differential Diagnosis") is a benign condition that will resolve with conservative measures and does not require imaging studies [9]. In fact, early imaging (before 6 weeks) has been shown to increase healthcare costs without providing any clear evidence of clinical benefit. Furthermore, routine imaging in these situations has the potential to produce harm by exposure to radiation and/or additional unnecessary interventions [10]. The following tables from the American College of Radiology provide clinical scenarios that warrant imaging and specify which imaging tests are most appropriate for each scenario:

Scenario 1 Acute, subacute, or chronic uncomplicated low back pain or radiculopathy. One or more of the following: low velocity trauma, osteoporosis, elderly individual, or chronic steroid use

Radiologic procedure	Rating[a]	Comments
X-ray lumbar spine	7	Initial study of choice especially in setting of osteoporosis or osteoporosis risk factors
CT lumbar spine without contrast	7	If suspicion for fracture is high and X-ray is negative
MRI lumbar spine without contrast	7	Can evaluate for ligamentous injury or in setting of worsening neuro deficit
Tc-99m bone scan with SPECT spine	3	Can uncover radiographically occult fractures
CT lumbar spine with contrast	3	
CT lumbar spine with/without contrast	1	
X-ray myelography and post-myelography CT lumbar spine	1	
X-ray discography and post-discography CT lumbar spine	1	

[a] Rating scale: 1, 2, and 3 usually not appropriate; 4, 5, and 6 may be appropriate; 7, 8, and 9 usually appropriate

Scenario 2 Acute, subacute, or chronic low back pain or radiculopathy. One or more of the following: suspicion of cancer, infection, or immunosuppression

Radiologic procedure	Rating[a]	Comments
MRI lumbar spine with/without contrast	8	Contrast helps for cancer patients suspected of epidural or intraspinal disease
MRI lumbar spine without contrast	7	Sufficient if low risk of epidural or intraspinal disease
CT lumbar spine with contrast	6	If MRI is contraindicated
CT lumbar spine without contrast	6	If MRI is contraindicated
X-ray lumbar spine	5	
Tc-99m bone scan with SPECT spine	4	Helps with anatomic localization if widespread metastasis is suspected
FDG-PET/CT whole body	4	Can help distinguish benign from malignant compression fractures but MRI is better
CT lumbar spine with/without contrast	3	If MRI is contraindicated
X-ray myelography and post-myelography CT lumbar spine	3	If MRI is contraindicated can be useful for anatomic localization and problem-solving

[a] Rating scale: 1, 2, and 3 usually not appropriate; 4, 5, and 6 may be appropriate; 7, 8, and 9 usually appropriate

Scenario 3 Acute, subacute, or chronic low back pain or radiculopathy. Surgery or intervention candidate with persistent or progressive symptoms during or following 6 weeks of conservative management

Radiologic procedure	Rating[a]	Comments
MRI lumbar spine without contrast	8	
CT lumbar spine with contrast	5	If MRI is contraindicated
CT lumbar spine without contrast	5	If MRI is contraindicated
MRI lumbar spine with/without contrast	5	If MRI without contrast is nondiagnostic or if history of prior lumbar surgery
X-ray lumbar spine	4	Usually not sufficient by itself but can help with surgical planning
Tc-99m bone scan with SPECT spine	4	Useful for facet arthropathy or stress fracture
X-ray discography and post-discography CT lumbar spine	3	Controversial but may be helpful in patients with pain >3 months

[a] Rating scale: 1, 2, and 3 usually not appropriate; 4, 5, and 6 may be appropriate; 7, 8, and 9 usually appropriate

Scenario 4 Low back pain or radiculopathy. New or progressing symptoms or clinical findings with history of prior lumbar surgery

Radiologic procedure	Rating[a]	Comments
MRI lumbar spine with/without contrast	8	Can differentiate disk from scar
CT lumbar spine with contrast	6	Useful in postfusion patients or when MRI is contraindicated or nondiagnostic
CT lumbar spine without contrast	6	Useful in postfusion patients or when MRI is contraindicated or nondiagnostic

Radiologic procedure	Rating[a]	Comments
MRI lumbar spine without contrast	6	Contrast is usually necessary
X-ray myelography and post-myelography CT lumbar spine	5	
X-ray lumbar spine	5	Flexion and extension views can be helpful
Tc-99m bone scan with SPECT spine	5	Helps detect and localize painful pseudarthrosis
X-ray discography and post-discography CT lumbar spine	5	
CT lumbar spine with/without contrast	3	

[a] Rating scale: 1, 2, and 3 usually not appropriate; 4, 5, and 6 may be appropriate; 7, 8, and 9 usually appropriate

Scenario 5 Low back pain with suspected cauda equina syndrome or rapidly progressive neurologic deficit

Radiologic procedure	Rating[a]	Comments
MRI lumbar spine without contrast	9	Use of contrast depends on clinical circumstances
MRI lumbar spine with/without contrast	8	Use of contrast depends on clinical circumstances
X-ray myelography and post-myelography CT lumbar spine	6	If MRI is contraindicated or nondiagnostic
CT lumbar spine with contrast	5	
CT lumbar spine without contrast	5	
X-ray lumbar spine	3	
CT lumbar spine with/without contrast	3	
Tc-99m bone scan with SPECT spine	2	

[a] Rating scale: 1, 2, and 3 usually not appropriate; 4, 5, and 6 may be appropriate 7, 8, and 9 usually appropriate

22.6 Introduction to Treatment

While developing a comprehensive pain management strategy in an ED setting is likely to be unrealistic, the proper use of counseling and the prescribing of appropriate short-term pain medications is an important aspect of patient care and can help eliminate repeat visits to the ED. The treatment of complicated back pain due to serious underlying etiologies requires appropriate subspecialty consultation and is beyond the scope of this chapter; however, the majority of back complaints do not fall into this category. The following section provides guidance on both non-pharmacologic and pharmacologic approaches to treatment:

- Patient education [4]
  - Reassure patients that acute back pain/radiculopathy is very common.

  - Around 50–75% of the time, acute back pain/radiculopathy resolves spontaneously by 4 weeks.
  - Around 90% of the time, acute back pack pain/radiculopathy resolves spontaneously by 6 weeks.
  - Majority of patients with acute back pain/radiculopathy do not require surgery even when there is an acute disk herniation present.
- Activity level
  - Avoid bed rest and return to regular activities as tolerated as soon as possible. Patients who return to normal activity have less pain and better functional recovery [11].
- Monitored exercise program
  - Evidence indicates only modest improvements in patients with chronic rather than acute back pain [12].
- Other physical modalities
  - Lack of evidence supporting electrical nerve stimulation, traction, ultrasound, interferential therapy, or short-wave diathermy—although all are considered safe.
  - Superficial heat application has some benefit in acute low back pain [13].
- NSAIDs [14]
  - Examples include ibuprofen, naproxen, meloxicam, ketorolac, and diclofenac.
  - Effective for short-term relief of acute and chronic low back pain.
  - No specific NSAID is clearly superior to another.
  - Cox-2 inhibitors have fewer GI side effects; however, they should be used cautiously in patients with cardiovascular disease.
  - Use all NSAIDs cautiously in patients with history of renal impairment or peptic ulcer disease.
  - Common side effects include GI upset and rash.
- Acetaminophen
  - As effective as NSAIDs for acute low back pain and perhaps less effective in chronic low back pain [14]
  - Can be used as adjunctive therapy along with NSAIDs
  - Less renal and GI toxicity than NSAIDs
  - Caution in hepatic impairment
- Skeletal muscle relaxants [15]
  - Examples include cyclobenzaprine, tizanidine, methocarbamol, and baclofen.
  - Considered second-line treatment or as an adjunctive to NSAIDs or acetaminophen.
  - Evidence does support their effectiveness in nonspecific acute low back pain over placebo.
  - No specific muscle relaxant is clearly superior to another.
  - Work best within 1–2 weeks of presentation.
  - Use with caution in the elderly due to increased risk of falls.
  - Common side effects include sedation and dry mouth.
- Opioids
  - Examples include hydrocodone, oxycodone, morphine, and codeine.

  - No clear evidence of benefit over NSAIDs or acetaminophen in acute back pain [16].
  - Should be reserved for patients with severe acute back pain who have failed first- or second-line treatments.
  - Only short courses should be prescribed in the acute setting.
  - May have some benefit for chronic back pain in select populations.
  - Common side effects include sedation, constipation, nausea, and addiction.
- Anticonvulsants
  - Examples include gabapentin, pregabalin, and carbamazepine.
  - Some evidence of benefits for patients with acute or chronic radiculopathy [16].
  - Common side effects include sedation and dizziness.
- Corticosteroids
  - Examples include prednisone and Solu-Medrol.
  - No evidence of any benefit in acute or chronic back pain [16].
  - Extensive side effect profile.

References

1. Murray CJ, Lopez AD. Measuring the global burden of disease. N Engl J Med. 2013;369(5):448–57.
2. Centers for Disease Control and Prevention. National Ambulatory Medical Care Survey: 2010 summary tables. Atlanta: Centers for Disease Control and Prevention; 2011. www.cdc.gov/nchs/data/ahcd/namcs_summary/2010_namcs_web_tables.pdf. Accessed 28 Dec 2015.
3. Martin BI, Deyo RA, Mirza SK, Turner JA, Comstock BA, Hollingworth W, et al. Expenditures and health status among adults with back and neck problems. JAMA. 2008;299:656–64.
4. Chou R, Cotton D, Rao JK, Taichman D, Williams S. In the clinic: low back pain. Ann Intern Med. 2014;160(11):ITC6–1.
5. Kinkade S. Evaluation and treatment of acute low back pain. Am Fam Physician. 2007;75(8):1181–8
6. Ombrect L. Disorders of the thoracic spine: pathology and treatment. In: A system of orthopedic medicine. 3rd ed. Churchill Livingstone, Elsevier; 2013. pp. E169–E184.
7. Vukmir RB. Drug seeking behavior. Am J Drug Alcohol Abuse. 2004;30(3):551–75.
8. Bickley LS, Szilagyi PG, Bates B. The musculoskeletal system. In Bates' guide to physical examination and history taking. 8th ed. Philadelphia: Lippincott Williams & Wilkins; 2003. p. 520–2.
9. American College of Radiology. ACR appropriateness criteria. Low back pain. Reston: American College of Radiology; 2015. https://acsearch.acr.org/docs/69483/Narrative/. Accessed 5 Dec 2015.
10. Chou R, Qaseem A, Owens DK, Shekelle P. Diagnostic imaging for low back pain: advice for high-value health care from the American College of Physicians. Ann Intern Med. 2011;154(3):181–9.
11. Hagen KB, Hilde G, Jamtvedt G, Winnem M. Bed rest for acute low-back pain and sciatica. Cochrane Database Syst Rev. 2004:CD001254.
12. Hayden JA, van Tulder MW, Malmivaara AV, Koes BW. Metaanalysis: exercise therapy for nonspecific low back pain. Ann Intern Med. 2005;142:765–75.

13. Chou R, Huffman LH, American Pain Society. Nonpharmacologic therapies for acute and chronic low back pain: a review of the evidence for an American Pain Society/American College of Physicians clinical practice guideline. Ann Intern Med. 2007;147:492–504.
14. Roelofs, PD, Deyo RA, Koes BW, Scholten RJ, van Tulder MW. Nonsteroidal anti-inflammatory drugs for low back pain. Cochrane Database Syst Rev. 2008:CD000396.
15. van Tulder MW, Touray T, Furlan AD, Solway S, Bouter LM. Muscle relaxants for non-specific low back pain. Cochrane Database Syst Rev. 2003:CD004252.
16. Chou R, Huffman LH, American Pain Society. Medications for acute and chronic low back pain: a review of the evidence for an American Pain Society/American College of Physicians clinical practice guideline. Ann Intern Med. 2007;147:505–14.

Nonemergency Skin Problems in the Emergency Department

23

James Medley

23.1 Introduction

3.3% of all emergency department visits were dermatologic conditions in a study from 2007 to 2015, with most of these representing cellulitis with or without abscess [1].

Infection is generally straightforward in ruling out (lack of significant pain, edema) and can be aided by imaging available in the ED including point-of-care ultrasound. Abscess, including paronychia and felon, is commonly treated in the ED as well, and it need not be further discussed here. Infectious treatment largely depends on body area and history, and outpatient management is usually sufficient. Primary care follow-up can be sought within a week of discharge.

Other common skin conditions such as acne vulgaris, rosacea, and pigment disorders such as vitiligo (patchy hypopigmentation), melasma (patchy hyperpigmentation), or cutaneous lesions (moles, etc.) can generally be evaluated to ensure that no bacterial or fungal component is present, treated if so, and discharged to primary care follow-up for further evaluation and treatment, which need not take place in the ED.

Table 23.1 demonstrates the distribution of skin-related diagnoses in ED visits during the same period. Most of these cases can certainly be managed in most primary care offices although urgent attention may be needed in some patients. Additionally, true dermatologic emergencies are quite rare, and discussion of them is beyond the scope of this text.

While most noninfectious skin neoplasms can certainly be evaluated through close outpatient follow-up, patients often experience significant distress when skin

J. Medley (✉)
Department of Community Health and Family Medicine, University of Florida College of Medicine, Gainesville, FL, USA
e-mail: jmed617@ufl.edu

B. K. Desai et al. (eds.), *Primary Care for Emergency Physicians*,
https://doi.org/10.1007/978-3-031-64676-8_23

Table 23.1 Diagnoses of skin conditions in ED visits [1]

	Cases (%)
Cellulitis and abscess—all sites	46.73
Rash and other nonspecific skin eruption	9.01
Dermatophytosis of nail	7.42
Neoplasm of uncertain behavior of skin	5.02
Contact dermatitis and other eczema unspecified cause	3.17
Urticaria unspecified	2.47
Herpes zoster without mention of complication	2.33
Benign neoplasm of skin of trunk except scrotum	2.24
Allergic urticaria	2.08
Unspecified local infection of skin and subcutaneous tissue	1.39
Onychia and paronychia of finger	1.05

Nadkarni et al. [1]

conditions manifest in itching, when there are pigment changes, or if significant body surface area is affected, bringing them to the emergency department for evaluation. This chapter thus focuses on such cases to aid the emergency clinician in deciding what treatment may be best until outpatient follow-up can be arranged.

23.2 Topical Glucocorticoids

In general, topical glucocorticoids are very useful in itching skin conditions as vehicles often act as emollients and cessation of inflammation and itching can be helpful to avoid scratching.

Topical steroids are classified according to potency, with class 1 glucocorticoids being "super-potent" and generally not appropriate for sensitive skin areas including the face, genitals, and axillae and class 7 glucocorticoids being mild, often available over the counter. Class 7 glucocorticoids may not be potent enough for thicker skin areas such as the back, palms, soles, and thighs. Recall that the vehicle affects potency, with ointments generally being more potent than cream at the same concentration and creams being more potent than lotions. Gels, solutions, and foams can be variable in potency.

In general, delicate and intertriginous skin should be managed with mild-moderately potent agents (classes 4–7), and decision should be based on skin thickness and degree of inflammation. A small prescription with close outpatient follow-up is recommended by this author.

In general, this author recommends becoming familiar with an agent per class to allow for fast medical decision-making based on the patient's presenting symptoms. Table 23.2 [2] shows suggested agents.

Table 23.2 Examples of widely available topical glucocorticoids, by class

Topical steroid class	Selected examples
Class 1 (super-potent)	Clobetasol propionate all vehicles 0.05% Fluocinonide cream 0.1%
Class 2 (high potency)	Clobetasol propionate 0.025% Fluocinonide cream, gel, ointment, solution 0.05%
Class 3 (high potency)	Triamcinolone acetonide 0.5% Fluocinonide cream 0.05% Betamethasone valerate foam 0.12%, ointment 0.1%
Class 4 (medium potency)	Hydrocortisone valerate ointment 0.2% Triamcinolone acetonide cream or ointment 0.1%, ointment 0.05%
Class 5 (low-medium potency)	Desonide gel, ointment 0.05% Hydrocortisone butyrate 0.1% Triamcinolone acetonide 0.025% ointment, 0.1% lotion
Class 6 (low potency)	Triamcinolone lotion, cream 0.025% Desonide foam, lotion, cream 0.05%
Class 7 (least potent)	1–2% Hydrocortisone including hydrocortisone acetate lotion, cream, ointment, gel, spray

U.S. Food and Drug Administration [2]

23.3 Eczematous Eruptions

23.3.1 Xerosis (Dry Skin) [3–9]

Dry skin presents typically as itching skin and tends to affect the extremities as exposure to humidity and other chemicals (e.g., harsh cleansers) tends to increase the risk of skin drying. Scale is typically very fine and powdery, if present, and skin can be faintly erythematous with cracking varying from fine, minute cracks to large cracks that can expose dermal vasculature and cause bleeding with minor trauma.

Risk factors include older age, decreased environmental relative humidity, cold weather, and underlying skin conditions. Diagnosis is typically clinical with no biopsy, imaging, or lab work needed.

Treatment includes avoiding exposure to cold or dry areas (humidifiers) and emollients, particularly those with slightly lower pH as this can inhibit skin enzymes that promote breakdown. Avoiding rough clothing, exposure to hot water or prolonged water exposure, and topical drying agents such as rubbing alcohol can also be helpful. Oatmeal baths can be helpful if water is not too hot, which can lead to excessive drying.

Medications such as topical steroids depending on body location and oral antihistamines such as hydroxyzine can be helpful in short courses to help relieve itching, which can perpetuate symptoms.

23.3.2 Atopic Dermatitis (Eczema)

This typically presents as an itch which develops a rash after consistent scratching by the patient; thus, it is commonly described as "the itch that rashes." Genetic factors likely play a role as twin concordance is high, 80%, compared to nonidentical siblings (20%), so a family history of eczema may be helpful in diagnosis [10, 11]. Additionally, it is associated with environmental allergies and asthma, which if present increase the suspicion that a fitting clinical presentation can be attributed to eczema [12, 13].

Presentation is highly variable, with age, skin tone, and duration since symptom onset playing a role in skin appearance. Intense itching and dry skin are nearly universal [14]. Skin can appear red, crusted, and scaly with crusting present if skin disruption leads to serous exudate. Older children and adults commonly present with rash to flexor surfaces of wrists, ankles, fossae (antecubital, popliteal), and hands. Early diagnosis is common, with nearly 85% of patients diagnosed before age 5.

Biopsy is not typically needed for the diagnosis but can be arranged by the primary care physician if initial treatment is not helpful by the time follow-up is arranged, preferably within 2 weeks (the recommended duration of a course of topical glucocorticoid medication).

Treatment is similar to xerosis, with emollients, environmental changes, and topical steroids based on the body location affected. Oral steroids are rarely needed.

23.3.3 Contact Dermatitis

Anyone can be affected by contact dermatitis, but as a delayed hypersensitivity reaction, it requires previous exposure to the agent in question and usually 48–72 h from exposure to eruption of symptoms. Nickel is the most common metal triggering contact dermatitis, while in North America, most cases are caused by exposure to urushiol-bearing plants including poison ivy, poison oak, and poison sumac [15].

The presentation is typically of intense pruritus followed by a sharply demarcated, often notably patterned (look for streaks, scratch marks from spreading exposure, or unusual shapes such as rectangles as clues to an external cause) erythematous rash often with excoriation, crusting from serous exudate, and skin breakdown in moderate-to-severe cases.

Treatment includes removing the offending stimulus (jewelry, buckles, contaminated clothing, chemicals), irrigation if contaminant may be present on the skin, and topical corticosteroids matched to body location. Note that the treatment may require up to 4 weeks of therapy for resolution of the underlying hypersensitivity mechanism [16]. Restoration of the skin barrier with moisturizers or emollients can be helpful as well.

23.3.4 Seborrheic Dermatitis

In this condition, skin inflammation is induced by yeast of the *Malassezia* species that feeds on phospholipids in the epidermis generally expressed after puberty (or in infants due to the action of maternal androgens in utero). Thus, the presentation is typically of itchy, flaky, red-yellow patches often described as "greasy" in areas bearing high sebum content, such as the scalp, nasolabial areas, and hair-bearing facial skin. Chest involvement is also described [17, 18].

If the clinical picture is uncertain, a skin scraping examined after treatment with 10% KOH solution often reveals yeast structures upon microscopy. Biopsy or fungal culture is not typically necessary for diagnosis.

Treatment is generally aimed at reducing the yeast population, as it is ubiquitous and thus cannot be eliminated, as well as reducing inflammation in moderate-to-severe acute cases to relieve symptoms. In general, ketoconazole 2% wash or creams and selenium-containing washes with gentle facial glucocorticoids such as desonide can be helpful. Advanced treatments, such as topical calcineurin inhibitors, can likely be deferred to primary care follow-up.

23.3.5 Urticaria

It is worth mentioning here that urticaria, or hives, often presents spontaneously without a clear trigger. These intensely itchy salmon-pink plaques can present anywhere on the body but usually erupt in higher temperature areas and areas of friction.

Exam for urticaria is usually straightforward. Lesions evolve over time, and often the exact pattern of lesions is different after a few minutes of re-evaluation.

Dermatographism, or an urticarial eruption in response to a light scratch on the skin, often allows a confident diagnosis of urticaria but is not always present.

After evaluation and elimination of concern for anaphylaxis, urticaria can be treated with high-dose antihistamines such as fexofenadine 360–720 mg daily, usually in two divided doses, with close primary care follow-up.

23.4 Parasite and Infestation Reactions

23.4.1 Scabies

In scabies, the mite *Sarcoptes scabiei* burrows under the top layers of skin, depositing eggs and fecal material which triggers the hypersensitivity reaction responsible for intense pruritus of the condition. The scabies mite is transmissible, sometimes even through fomites (such as clothing), but prolonged contact is generally needed for transmission to occur.

Common sites of infestation include web spaces, flexural points, genitalia, periareolar breast, waist, and umbilicus. It is rare for only one site to be involved [19, 20]. An intensely itchy erythematous papule in a common body area should prompt suspicion of scabies, and if a burrow (a gray-to-red serpiginous line in the skin) is present, a skin scraping (with a scalpel or curette) may reveal mites or eggs on microscopy with KOH preparation. While 100% specific, a negative test should not eliminate the possibility of scabies as sensitivity is relatively low, less than 40% [21].

Treatment includes eliminating organisms in the skin as well as environmental sources to prevent reinfestation. 5% Permethrin cream applied neck-to-feet for 8–12 h prior to rinsing is preferred. It is important to stress that all skin creases, web spaces, and folds need to have cream applied in a thin coat. If permethrin is unsuccessful or cannot be applied, systemic ivermectin therapy is preferred [22]. This is weight based; consult a pharmacist or dosing calculator, but the typical dose is 200 mcg/kg given once with a one-week repeat dose. Clothing, bedding, and towels should be washed with hot water and dried on high heat. Soft toys can be placed in a plastic bag and sealed for 2 weeks if drying is not feasible [22].

23.4.2 Bedbugs [22]

The bite of bedbugs, most often *Cimex lectularius*, is often very similar to other arthropod bites, with reactions to bites possible. The typical "breakfast, lunch, and dinner" arrangement of linear bites is common but is not specific to bedbugs (fleas are another common cause of this pattern). Bites occur at night, but reactions to bites can continue to form throughout the day. Look for bites in exposed areas as they generally do not climb under clothing.

Treatment is often targeted at reactions including body-specific topical steroids, treatment of skin infections, and investigating any clinical concern for bloodborne pathogens.

Household eradication can be attempted with steam treatments and heat treatments, but consultation with a pest infestation professional is generally recommended.

23.4.3 Pediculosis (Lice) [22]

Lice infestations are most commonly of the head lice variety, *Pediculus humanus capitis*, a different species from the body louse, which can transmit disease including Rickettsial infection.

Generally, pruritus of the scalp is the presenting symptom, and lice are often easy to find for diagnostic confirmation. Eggs, or nits, are generally found affixed to hair shafts and can be quite small, around 0.5 mm in diameter, and range from white to brown. Without visualization of lice or nits, consider scalp eczema, seborrheic dermatitis, and even scalp psoriasis in the differential.

Transmission is generally from head-to-head contact with another infected individual, but fomite spread (hats, combs, pillows) is possible.

Many common treatments exist including attempting to suffocate lice and nits with products such as petrolatum and mayonnaise. These generally are less effective than pharmacologic treatments although they may soften nits and aid in removal with a **nit comb**, which is necessary to prevent reinfection with a new generation of lice.

Permethrin 1% cream rinse (available OTC) is applied after shampooing and left for 10 min prior to rinsing. A repeat treatment in 7–10 days is recommended. Nit combing is necessary to remove nits and prevent hatching.

There is no need to withhold children from school due to lice. Close contacts should be examined or notified, and combs should be sanitized by placing in hot water.

23.5 Fungal Disorders

23.5.1 Dermatophytes, "Tinea" [22]

Dermatophyte fungi can infiltrate superficial layers of the epidermis when organisms are exposed to open areas of skin (abrasions, etc.) from fomites and direct contact. Lesions are generally noticed visually as itching is mild if present at all. Lesions are generally round, though they need not be perfectly circular or oval. The peripheral areas of lesions are generally the most active (i.e., most raised, most erythematous, and scale is usually concentrated), as the fungal organisms progress from the initial inoculation point and outwards as they consume epidermal nutrients. In larger lesions, the center may even appear normal.

Dermatophyte nail involvement causes separation of laminated keratin layers forming the nail, often with fungal debris deposited in the new space, creating a thickened, opacified nail. Early involvement is noted by white opacification, and prolonged involvement often leads to nail discoloration (gray, yellow).

Diagnosis is often easily made with a potassium hydroxide 10% preparation of a skin scraping viewed under a microscope slide with hyphal elements visualized.

The location of the lesion determines the name, and often treatment; see the table below.

Topical terbinafine 1% cream is generally preferred, with clotrimazole cream also being appropriate.

Oral therapy includes micro-griseofulvin at 20 mg/kg per day for children and oral terbinafine 250 mg daily in adults. Tinea capitis often requires 6 weeks of therapy. Widespread tinea corporis typically resolves with 2 weeks of therapy.

Onychomycosis, or nail dermatophytosis, requires a prolonged course of oral therapy. Patients can be reassured, provided with topical medications for any skin involvement, and referred to primary care for further management.

Scalp *Tinea capitis*	Systemic	10 days
Facial hair *Tinea barbae*	Systemic likely	10 days
Body *Tinea corporis, "ringworm"*	Topical Systemic in widespread or difficult areas	Apply topical treatment for 2 days after resolution (can be up to 4 weeks)
Genitalia *Tinea cruris, "jock itch"*	Topical	Same as above
Toes and web spaces *Tinea pedis, "athlete's foot"*	Topical	Same as above

Tinea versicolor, often affecting individuals starting at puberty, can be widespread and does not display a classic round shape, but "active borders" with scale and even pigment changes in the skin should prompt the KOH skin scraping, which in this case yields the "spaghetti and meatball" appearance of hyphae and yeast buds. Treatment is generally to control the ubiquitous fungal organism (*Malassezia furfur*) as cure is not possible, with topical ketoconazole shampoo applied for 5 min twice weekly while bathing, and then thoroughly rinsing.

23.5.2 Candidiasis, Intertrigo [22]

This is a superficial infection of skin caused by *Candida* species typically introduced through trauma, often microtrauma such as skin maceration and breakdown (thus, presence in skin folds or flexural areas is very common) or abrasions (high-friction areas). In infants and toddlers, this often presents in the diaper area as "diaper rash."

The rash is often painless although irritation or itching can occur. Spread to other areas can occur through scratching.

Exam usually shows "beefy red" rash with mild skin edema that may cause the rash to be somewhat elevated over the surrounding skin. Lesions called "satellite lesions," essentially erythematous papules scattered beyond the periphery of the main lesion, are often present. These represent eruptions of new areas of infection, often involving hair follicles. These need not be present for a diagnosis. Wood lamp examination can be helpful to rule out *erythrasma*, a bacterial skin infection that can appear very similar to candidiasis but with red fluorescence (with no fluorescence in candidiasis).

Treatment of *erythrasma* is with erythromycin preferably, while candidiasis can be treated with topical preparations until the rash is gone, typically twice daily for 1–2 weeks. Agents include azoles (ketoconazole, clotrimazole) or nystatin. Nystatin ointment has the added benefit of acting as a barrier to friction allowing the normal skin barrier to heal and protect against future infection. Nystatin powder is available to help in high-moisture areas. Systemic treatment with fluconazole is rarely needed except when high body surface area involvement makes topical treatment inconvenient, but can be done with 150 mg oral doses once weekly for 4 weeks. Use weight-based dosing for individuals <50 kg.

23.6 Closing Remarks

There are, of course, nearly infinite causes of various rashes ranging from mild and harmless to clinically significant due to reflection of underlying disease (e.g., petechiae), dangerous because of the risk of complications (e.g., large skin bullae or erythema multiforme), or critical (e.g., high-surface-area skin sloughing).

Naturally, the latter examples often require emergency treatment such as hydration, stabilization, or treatment with medications for infection. The emergency physician is thus more occupied by preservation of life or limb by these presentations, and the rash, if persistent, can be assessed later when the patient is stable. If a rash is a mimicker of infection, empiric treatment and follow-up with primary care for possible biopsy or referral can help distinguish the cause.

References

1. Nadkarni A, Dormeisen N, Hill D, Feldman SR. The most common dermatology diagnoses in the emergency department. 2016. JAAD.org. https://www.jaad.org/article/S0190-9622(16)30606-5/fulltext. Accessed 17 Aug 2022.
2. U.S. Food and Drug Administration. Approved drug products with therapeutic equivalence (Orange Book). https://www.accessdata.fda.gov/scripts/cder/ob/default.cfm. Accessed 18 June 2017.
3. Yosipovitch G, Bernhard JD. Clinical practice. Chronic pruritus. N Engl J Med. 2013;368:1625.
4. White-Chu EF, Reddy M. Dry skin in the elderly: complexities of a common problem. Clin Dermatol. 2011;29:37.
5. Boccanfuso SM, Cosmet L, Volpe AR, Bensel A. Skin xerosis. Clinical report on the effect of a moisturizing soap bar. Cutis. 1978;21:703.
6. Abbas S, Goldberg JW, Massaro M. Personal cleanser technology and clinical performance. Dermatol Ther. 2004;17(Suppl 1):35.
7. Steinhoff M, Neisius U, Ikoma A, et al. Proteinase-activated receptor-2 mediates itch: a novel pathway for pruritus in human skin. J Neurosci. 2003;23:6176.
8. Lodén M. The clinical benefit of moisturizers. J Eur Acad Dermatol Venereol. 2005;19:672.
9. Draelos ZD. Active agents in common skin care products. Plast Reconstr Surg. 2010;125:719.
10. Larsen FS, Holm NV, Henningsen K, Atopic dermatitis. A genetic-epidemiologic study in a population-based twin sample. J Am Acad Dermatol. 1986;15:487.
11. Schultz LF. Atopic dermatitis: a genetic-epidemiologic study in a population-based twin sample. J Am Acad Dermatol. 1993;28:719.
12. von Kobyletzki LB, Bornehag CG, Hasselgren M, et al. Eczema in early childhood is strongly associated with the development of asthma and rhinitis in a prospective cohort. BMC Dermatol. 2012;12:11.
13. Bantz SK, Zhu Z, Zheng T. The atopic march: progression from atopic dermatitis to allergic rhinitis and asthma. J Clin Cell Immunol. 2014;5:202.
14. Rudikoff D, Lebwchl M. Atopic dermatitis. Lancet. 1998;351:1715
15. Zug KA, Warshaw EM, Fowler JF Jr, et al. Patch-test results of the North American Contact Dermatitis Group 2005-2006. Dermatitis. 2009;20:149.
16. Bikowski JB. Hand eczema: diagnosis and management. Cutis. 2008;82:9.
17. Faergemann J, Bergbrant IM, Dohsé M, et al. Seborrhoeic dermatitis and Pityrosporum (Malassezia) folliculitis: characterization of inflammatory cells and mediators in the skin by immunohistochemistry. Br J Dermatol. 2001;144:549.
18. Riciputo RM, Oliveri S, Micali G, Sapuppo A. Phospholipase activity in Malassezia furfur pathogenic strains. Mycoses. 1996;39:233.
19. Pomares C, Marty P, Delaunay P. Isolated itching of the genitals. Am J Trop Med Hyg. 2014;90:589.
20. Eshagh K, DeKlotz CM, Friedlander SF. Infant with a papular eruption localized to the back. JAMA Pediatr. 2014;168:379.
21. Micheletti RG, Dominguez AR, Wanat KA. Bedside diagnostics in dermatology: Parasitic and noninfectious diseases. J Am Acad Dermatol. 2017;77:221.
22. Krowchuk DP, Mancini AJ. Pediatric dermatology: a quick reference guide. Section on Dermatology, American Academy of Pediatrics; 2012.

Anxiety

24

Christopher Wallace and Brooke Taylor

24.1 Introduction

Generalized anxiety disorder (GAD) and panic disorder have a 12-month prevalence in US adults aged 18–64 of 2.9% and a lifetime prevalence of 7.7% and 4.6% in women and men, respectively [1]. GAD can be difficult to diagnose even in the primary care setting. The setting of the emergency department lends itself to an increased difficulty of diagnosis due to symptom presentations that mirror GAD, including headaches, abdominal pain, and shortness of breath. Diagnostic criteria for GAD as defined by the American Psychiatric Association in DSM 5 can be found in Table 24.1.

It is important to note that the diagnosis of GAD does not apply when the clinical picture can better be attributed to another psychiatric diagnosis, medical condition, substance use, or substance withdrawal [1].

People with GAD have excessive anxiety about typical, everyday situations. These patients may have a range of complaints including, but not limited to, sleep disturbances, restlessness, muscular tension, gastrointestinal complaints, and chronic headaches [1].

Panic disorder is defined as recurrent, unexpected panic attacks for more than 1 month in association with at least one of the following symptoms: persistent concern about having additional attacks, worry about the attacks' implications or consequences, or a significant change in behavior as a result of the attacks. Panic disorder is also a diagnosis of exclusion and cannot be better explained by another medical condition, substance use, or other psychiatric condition [2]. Comorbid axis disorders, such as major depressive disorder or general anxiety disorder, are commonly associated with panic disorder [3]. In addition, panic disorder is associated with low education and relatively low probability of working full time [3].

C. Wallace (✉) · B. Taylor
University of Central Florida, Orlando, FL, USA

B. K. Desai et al. (eds.), *Primary Care for Emergency Physicians*,
https://doi.org/10.1007/978-3-031-64676-8_24

Table 24.1 DSM 5—generalized anxiety disorder criteria

(a) Excessive anxiety and worry (apprehensive expectation), occurring more days than not for at least 6 months, about a number of events or activities (such as work or school performance)
(b) The person finds it difficult to control the worry
(c) The anxiety and worry are associated with three (or more) of the following six symptoms (with at least some symptoms present for more days than not for the past 6 months). Note: Only one item is required in children. 1. Restlessness or feeling keyed up or on edge 2. Being easily fatigued 3. Difficulty concentrating or mind going blank 4. Irritability 5. Muscle tension 6. Sleep disturbance (difficulty falling or staying asleep or restless unsatisfying sleep)
(d) The focus of the anxiety and worry is not confined to features of an axis I disorder, e.g., the anxiety or worry is not about having a panic attack (as in panic disorder), being embarrassed in public (as in social phobia), being contaminated (as in obsessive-compulsive disorder), being away from home or close relatives (as in separation anxiety disorder), gaining weight (as in anorexia nervosa), having multiple physical complaints (as in somatization), or having a serious illness (as in hypochondriasis), and the anxiety and worry do not occur exclusively during post-traumatic stress disorder
(e) The anxiety, worry, or physical symptoms cause clinically significant distress or impairment in social, occupational, or other important areas of functioning
(f) The disturbance is not due to the direct physiological effects of a substance (e.g., a drug of abuse, a medication) or a general medical condition (e.g., hyperthyroidism) and does not occur exclusively during a mood disorder, a psychotic disorder, or a pervasive developmental disorder

It is thought that anxiety is often a learned response to noxious or aversive stimuli [4]. Patients suffering from an anxiety disorder are more likely to have other medical issues and longer hospital stays, undergo more procedures, incur higher healthcare costs, suffer from failure at school or work, have lower-paying jobs, and are more often financially dependent on welfare [4]. In addition, anxiety disorders are the most prevalent mental disorder among American children and adolescents [5].

Identification of generalized anxiety disorder is of special importance to clinicians in both the emergent and non-emergent settings, because misdiagnosis can lead to costly, invasive, and/or harmful unnecessary medical testing.

24.2 Risk Factors for Anxiety

- A genetic component plays a role in anxiety disorders:
  - The greatest association is in panic disorder, generalized anxiety disorder, and phobias.
- Having involved, controlling, and rejecting parents.
- Female.
- Low education.

- Low socioeconomic status.
- Social disability.
- Family history of anxiety disorders.
- Introverted personality in early childhood.
- Traumatic life events.
- Sleep disturbances.
- Poor physical health.

24.3 Differential Diagnosis

Anxiety is a diagnosis of exclusion. A thorough medical evaluation is needed to both rule out and alleviate the patient's concern for serious medical conditions.

- Medication side effects
  - Beta agonists
  - Caffeine
  - Digoxin toxicity
  - Levodopa
  - Nicotinic acid
  - SSRIs
  - Steroids
  - Stimulants
  - Theophylline
  - Synthetic thyroid hormone
- Cardiovascular
  - Acute coronary syndrome
  - Congestive heart failure
  - Mitral valve prolapse
  - Dysrhythmias
  - Syncope
  - Hypertension
- Pulmonary
  - Asthma
  - Chronic obstructive pulmonary disease
  - Hyperventilation
  - Pneumonia
  - Pneumothorax
  - Pulmonary edema
  - Pulmonary embolus
- Endocrine
  - Hyperthyroidism
  - Hypothyroidism
  - Hyperadrenalism
- Gastrointestinal

  - Gastroesophageal reflux disease
  - Irritable bowel syndrome
  - Colitis
    Typically of a chronic nature
  - Ulcers
- Neoplastic
  - Carcinoid syndrome
  - Pheochromocytoma
  - Insulinoma
- Neurologic
  - Parkinsonism
  - Encephalopathy
  - Restless leg syndrome
  - Seizure
  - Vertigo
  - Brain tumor
- Psychiatric
  - Affective disorders
  - Panic disorder
  - Agoraphobia
  - Conduct disorder
  - Social anxiety disorder
  - Post-traumatic stress disorder
  - Illness anxiety disorder
  - Prolonged grief disorder
  - Bipolar disorders
  - Personality disorders
  - Oppositional defiant disorder
  - Depression
  - Drug abuse
  - Drug dependence
  - Drug withdrawal
    Both illicit and prescribed
- Other conditions
  - Anaphylaxis
  - Anemia
    Typically chronic
  - Electrolyte abnormalities
    Occurring over time
  - Porphyria
  - Menopause

24.4 Types of Anxiety Disorders [3]

- Specific phobia
  - 18.4% prevalence
  - Fear or anxiety about a specific object or situation (i.e., swimming in the ocean)
- Social phobia
  - 13.0% prevalence
  - Fear or anxiety about one or more social situations where the individual is exposed to possible scrutiny by others
- Post-traumatic stress disorder
  - 10.1% prevalence.
  - Intrusive thoughts and flashbacks of traumatic events, avoidance of reminders, hypervigilance, and sleep disturbances lead to social and occupational dysfunction.
- Generalized anxiety disorder
  - 9.0% prevalence.
  - At least 6 months of persistent and excessive anxiety and worry occur on most days, with difficulty controlling the worry.
- Separation anxiety
  - 8.7% prevalence
  - Excessive anxiety or fear concerning separation from those to whom the individual is attached
- Panic disorder
  - 6.8% prevalence.
  - An abrupt surge of intense fear or discomfort that reaches a peak within minutes and can be recurrent and unexpected.
  - Dizziness, lightheadedness, tingling sensations, and fear of dying are common.
- Agoraphobia
  - 3.7% prevalence
  - Fear or anxiety about using public transportation, being in open or enclosed spaces, being in a crowd, or being outside alone
- Obsessive-compulsive disorder
  - 2.7% prevalence
  - Recurrent intrusive thoughts and urges, as well as repetitive mental and behavioral acts/compulsions that the individual feels driven to perform, leading to anxiety and distress

24.5 History

The patient's history plays a large part in the diagnosis of anxiety disorders. It is important to understand the timeline of worry and/or fear and elicit underlying causes for concern. Multiple negative workups for a concerning issue may indicate underlying anxiety. The Beck Anxiety Inventory (BAI) is a 21-question multiple-choice self-reported inventory, designed for pediatrics to geriatrics, that helps measure a patient's severity of anxiety [6]. The test can be used to establish a baseline level of anxiety as well as to better understand posttreatment outcomes. Unfortunately, this tool does not discriminate well between anxiety and depression [7].

24.6 Physical Exam

Physical exam may yield little in helping diagnose anxiety disorders, as there are many overlapping symptoms in signs with other disease states.

Organ system	Physical exam findings
CNS/PNS	• Dizziness • Paresthesia • Lightheadedness • Sweating • Clammy hands
Cardiovascular	• Palpitations • Tachycardia • Flushing • Pallor • Hot and cold spells
Respiratory	• Hyperventilation • SOB • Chest constriction/tightness
Gastrointestinal	• Dry mouth • Diarrhea • Upset stomach • Feelings of a lump in the throat • Nausea • Vomiting
Urinary	• Frequent urination
Musculoskeletal	• Muscle tightness/spasm • Back pain • Tremors • Headache • Weakness • Fatigue • Restlessness

24.7 Labs and Imaging

Laboratory tests are typically only useful in ruling out other medical conditions. A complete blood count, electrolyte panel (including glucose, creatinine, and calcium), liver panel, urine drug screen, and thyroid function tests may be useful in certain circumstances. Imaging is only necessary to interrogate lab abnormalities and rule out organic disease. Imaging can help to lessen patient concerns about physical pathologies.

24.8 Introduction to Treatment

There are several modalities aimed at treating anxiety disorders. These include education, psychotherapy, and pharmacotherapy. Combination therapy is often needed; however, any necessary treatment that is needed in addition to the acute phase warrants a psychiatric consultation. A careful history should help to elucidate the cause of a patient's anxiety. Any reversible causes should be treated accordingly. Medical conditions (i.e., hyperthyroidism) and medication side effects (i.e., theophylline toxicity) should be treated initially to see if anxiety resolves.

- Education
  - Patients should be counseled that anxiety is real and that they are not "crazy."
  - Providers should make patients aware of the different treatment modalities and refer them accordingly to appropriate services such as psychiatry, psychology, or other counseling resources.
- Psychotherapy
  - Behavioral therapy and cognitive behavioral therapy have been demonstrated to be the most efficacious types of psychotherapy.
  - Cognitive behavioral therapy has been shown as an efficacious and effective treatment for generalized anxiety disorder [8].
  - The outcome of treatment is determined by:
    - Severity of anxiety
    - Level of functioning before symptom onset
    - Motivation for treatment
    - Support system
    - Ability to comply with psychotherapy
- Pharmacotherapy
  - Considerations for medication management include:
    - Prescribing the lowest effective dose
    - Intermittent vs long-term pharmacotherapy
    - Quantity of medication being prescribed, especially out of the emergency department
    - Informing the patient of medication side effects and interactions

24.9 Pharmacologic Treatment

When considering treatment, providers should choose pharmacologic agents based on the type of anxiety they are trying to treat. They should take into consideration what diagnosis the patient has, whether their condition is acute or chronic, and determining if the benefits of the medication outweigh the side effects.

24.9.1 Antidepressant Agents

The first-line drug for the treatment of many anxiety disorders would be a selective serotonin reuptake inhibitor (SSRI). SSRIs are considered second-generation antidepressants and have a safer adverse event profile when compared to first-generation antidepressants like tricyclic antidepressants (TCAs) and monoamine oxidase inhibitors (MAOIs) [9].

(a) SSRIs

SSRI	Pitfall(s)
Fluoxetine	May initially cause anxiety
Paroxetine	Partially sedating
Citalopram	QT prolongation
Escitalopram	Fewer drug interactions
Sertraline	Decreased libido, failure to ejaculate

(b) Alpha-2 antagonist

Alpha-2 antagonist	Pitfall(s)
Mirtazapine	Sedating, increased appetite, and weight gain

24.9.2 Benzodiazepines

These medications are effective anxiolytics for acute anxiety. They are fast in onset and can provide immediate relief. It is acceptable for an emergency physician to prescribe a short course of benzodiazepines upon discharge to bridge the patient until they can be seen by a psychiatrist. However, it is not recommended to use benzodiazepines routinely as they are associated with central nervous system depression leading to fatigue, dizziness, increased reaction times, and impaired driving skills as well as a risk of developing a dependency on them. Due to these side effects, benzodiazepines are not recommended as a first-line treatment for anxiety disorders [10].

Selected benzodiazepines
Alprazolam
Clonazepam
Lorazepam

Pitfalls

- These drugs should not be used for chronic therapy due to their:
- Abuse potential
- Side effect profile
- Danger during withdrawal
- Severe side effects may include:
  - Anterograde amnesia
  - Daytime sleepiness
  - Decreased respiratory drive
- Stopping benzodiazepines suddenly can lead to:
  - Sleep disturbances
  - Irritability
  - Worsening anxiety
  - Panic attacks
  - Sweating
  - Confusion
  - Nausea
  - Hallucinations
  - Seizures
  - Psychosis
- Long-term benzodiazepine uses should be weaned rather than stopped suddenly to help prevent the life-threatening symptoms.

References

1. Locke AB, Kirst N, Schultz CG. Diagnosis and management of generalized anxiety disorder and panic disorder in adults. Am Fam Physician. 2015;91(9):617–24.
2. DeGeorge KC, Grover M, Streeter GS. Generalized anxiety disorder and panic disorder in adults. Am Fam Physician. 2022;106(2):157–64.
3. Tilli V, Suominem K, Karlsson H. Panic disorder in primary care: comorbic psychiatric disorders and their persistence. Scand J Prim Health Care. 2012;30(4):247–53. https://doi.org/10.3109/02813432.2012.732471. PMCID: PMC3520420.
4. Michels P, Steadman M. Anxiety disorders. In: Lebowitz H, editor. Current diagnosis & treatment: family medicine. 4th ed. New York: McGraw-Hill Education; 2015. p. 606–17.
5. Zarafshan H, Mohammadi M-R, Salmanian M. Prevalence of anxiety disorders among children and adolescents in Iran: a systematic review. Iran J Psychiatry. 2015;10(1):1–7. PubMed ID: 26005473.
6. Grant M. Beck anxiety inventory. http://webcache.googleusercontent.com/search?q=cache:F4qHbA5sI0MJ:www.manchester.gov.uk/download/downloads/id/19268/beck_anxiety_inventory_explanation.pdf+&cd=2&hl=en&ct=clnk&gl=us.
7. Muntingh AD, van der Feltz-Cornelis CM, van Marwijk HW, Spinhoven P, Penninx BW, van Balkom AJ. Is the beck anxiety inventory a good tool to assess the severity of anxiety? A primary care study in The Netherlands study of depression and anxiety (NESDA). BMC Fam Pract. 2011;12:66. https://doi.org/10.1186/1471-2296-12-66. PMID: PMC3224107.

8. Kaczkurkin AN, Foa EB. Cognitive-behavioral therapy for anxiety disorders: an update on the empirical evidence. Dialogues Clin Neurosci. 2015;17(3):337–46. https://doi.org/10.31887/DCNS.2015.17.3/akaczkurkin.
9. Yates W. Anxiety disorders. Medscape. 2015. http://emedicine.medscape.com/article/286227-overview. Accessed 14 Nov 2015.
10. Bandelow B, Michaelis S, Wedekind D. Treatment of anxiety disorders. Dialogues Clin Neurosci. 2017;19(2):93–107. https://doi.org/10.31887/DCNS.2017.19.2/bbandelow.

Depression

25

Christopher Wallace and Lucas Winter

25.1 Introduction

Depression affects more than 280 million people worldwide with the incidence increasing since the onset of the COVID-19 pandemic [1, 2]. It continues to be the leading cause of disability globally [3]. Depression-related chief complaints are common, constituting an estimated 11.4% of patients who present in the emergency department (ED) in the United States [4].

Despite the high prevalence, the presence of a depressive disorder may not be known. It is estimated up to 10% of patients who present in ambulatory settings have a depressive disorder and around half of these patients are undiagnosed [5]. These patients may present with psychosomatic symptoms in the ED, such as lower back pain or abdominal pain, masking the primary etiology. While recognition of depressive disorders in the ED or an ambulatory care clinic can be challenging due to the large volume of patients and high acuity of patients being seen, it is nonetheless important. Failure to recognize depressive disorders is a barrier to care; referring patients to appropriate treatment can save lives by prevention of suicide, improving quality of life for the patient and their family, and prevention of future unnecessary health-care visits [6, 7].

Major depressive disorder is associated with increased medical comorbidities, such as heart disease, diabetes, and stroke, which are thought to be related to a complex interplay of psychobiological factors [7]. These patients are more likely to suffer complications and present to the ED for these conditions [5, 7]. Patients with comorbid depression are also more likely to require admission to the hospital [4]. It is important to recognize the complexity of these patients.

C. Wallace · L. Winter (✉)
University of Central Florida, Orlando, FL, USA
e-mail: lucas.winter@hca.healthcare.com

B. K. Desai et al. (eds.), *Primary Care for Emergency Physicians*,
https://doi.org/10.1007/978-3-031-64676-8_25

25.2 Risk Factors

Lifetime prevalence of a major depressive episode is reported at around 16% for the general population in the United States [8]. Certain populations are known to be at an increased risk. Published risk factors for major depressive disorder include: [8–10]

- Female gender
- Middle age (45–64 years old)
- Multiple medical comorbidities
- Lack of social support
- Members of the LGBTQ community

For emergency providers, the principal goal in identifying major depressive disorder is to prevent depressed patients from harming themselves or others. The risk factors for major depression and suicidality do not necessarily coincide. For example, females are more likely to be depressed, but males are more likely to succeed in committing suicide [11].

The following factors are known to be linked with greater risk of suicide and should be taken into consideration when deciding whether or not to admit a patient for depression/suicidality [11, 12]:

- Repeated suicide attempts, which is the strongest predictive factor of suicide risk, especially if previous attempts were planned and lethal means were used
- Male gender
- Widowed, divorced, or separated individuals
- Relationship difficulties and conflicts
- Active unemployment
- Social isolation
- Lack of supportive family and friends
- Substance abuse
- Acute or chronic progressive illness
- Lack of insight into condition
- History of major depressive disorder, mood disorders, schizophrenia, or panic disorder
- Family history of suicide
- Lack of religious taboo against suicide
- Unstable or inappropriate affect

25.3 Diagnostic Criteria

The diagnosis of major depressive disorder requires a total of five of the listed criteria below. Anhedonia or depressed mood must be one of the criteria:

- Depressed mood

- Anhedonia
- Significant weight change or appetite change
- Insomnia or hypersomnia
- Psychomotor agitation or retardation
- Fatigue or loss of energy nearly every day
- Feelings of worthlessness
- Excessive or inappropriate guilt nearly every day
- Diminished ability to concentrate, or indecisiveness, nearly every day
- Recurrent thoughts of death and/or suicide

The symptoms must cause significant distress or impairment and may not be due to the direct physiological effects of a substance or general medical condition [13].

25.4 Differential Diagnosis

The differential diagnosis for major depressive disorder is broad and includes:

- Infection
  - HIV encephalopathy
  - Meningitis
  - Encephalitis
  - Lyme disease
- Substance abuse
  - Intoxication or withdrawal
- Medication side effects
  - Steroids
  - Antihypertensives
  - Hormone therapy
- Trauma
- Intracranial mass
- CNS disorders
  - Multiple sclerosis
  - Seizures
  - Alzheimer's disease
  - Microangiopathic lesions
- Metabolic disorders
  - Vitamin deficiencies: thiamine (B1), pyridoxine (B6), and cobalamin (B12)
- Endocrine disorders
  - Hypothyroidism
  - Cushing's syndrome
  - Hyperparathyroidism
  - Addison's disease
- Autoimmune disease
  - Systemic lupus erythematosus

- Obstructive sleep apnea
- Other psychiatric conditions
  - Complex bereavement
  - Bipolar depression
  - Schizoaffective disorder

25.5 History

Important clues from history known to increase a patient's likelihood of committing suicide include but are not limited to [14]:

- Feelings of hopelessness, helplessness, and guilt.
- Few or weak reasons to live.
- Suicidal ideations that are frequent, intense, prolonged, and pervasive.
- Patient with an unambiguous or continuing wish to die.
- Prior attempt.
- Suicide plan is realistic.
- Patient has access to firearms.
- Planned suicide includes a situation where rescue is unlikely.

25.6 Physical Exam

The diagnosis of major depressive disorder is usually made with a thorough history, but physical examination of a depressed patient remains an important adjunct. A comprehensive physical exam will help in the investigation of somatic complaints and in evaluating other potentially more emergent issues that may present with the chief complaint of depression (i.e., ingestion, intoxication).

One vital aspect of the physical exam is the mental status exam, which should include determination of:

- The patient's affect
- Appearance
- Orientation
- Attention
- Memory
- Speech pattern
- Level of consciousness
- Judgment
- Thought content

25.7 Red Flags

These physical exam red flags should alert you to consider more pressing diagnoses and consider medical/toxicologic explanations for a patient's depressed feelings:

- Abnormal vital signs
- Disorientation
- Clouded consciousness
- Focal neurologic deficits
- Recent memory loss in younger patients
- Signs of trauma

Patients with any of these findings warrant further workup. Helpful labs for these patients include [15]:

- Complete blood count
- Serum electrolytes
- Creatinine
- Hepatic enzymes
- Thyroid-stimulating hormone level + free T4
- Ethanol
- Urinalysis
- Pregnancy test
- Arterial blood gas
- Cerebrospinal fluid examination
- Electrocardiogram
- Computed tomography or magnetic resonance imaging of the brain
- Salicylate and acetaminophen levels in suicidal patients

25.8 Treatment

After properly recognizing a patient with major depressive disorder in the ED or in clinic, it can be challenging to provide proper treatment and disposition. An important first step is to stratify patients as high, moderate, or low risk for immediate harm to self and others.

High-risk patients are those who exhibit:

- Violent behaviors
- Agitation
- Endorse active suicidal or homicidal intent
- Require physical restraints
- Those who present after engaging in a possibly lethal suicide attempt (i.e., gunshot wound to the head or reported ingestion)

These patients require admission to a psychiatric facility for inpatient psychiatric therapy after medical clearance.

The following important steps should also be taken for all patients who are in the high-risk category:

- Disrobe, gown, and search the patient for potentially dangerous items.
- Determine if the patient needs to be detained for emergency evaluation.
- Treat medical conditions.
- Communication with the patient should be made while keeping the exit accessible for the provider, avoiding excessive eye contact, and using a nonthreatening voice.
- Enforce acceptable limits of behavior with the patient.

Any patient who is significantly agitated (shouting, cursing, threatening, physically aggressive, attempting to elope) or who is noncompliant with the established limits may require sedation and/or restraints. There is potential for harm to the patient with either sedation or restraints, so an effort should be made to de-escalate the situation verbally. If this is not successful, parenteral administration of sedation agents may be used. Benzodiazepines and antipsychotics (first and second generation) are considered first-line agents [16, 17]. Summary of the time to onset of sedation, dosing, and special considerations for benzodiazepines and antipsychotics are summarized in the table below.

The table shows parenteral medications used as first-line agents in acute agitation [17].

	Onset (min)	Initial dose (mg)	Considerations
Benzodiazepines			
Diazepam	30 min (IV)	5–10 mg (IV)	– Avoid IM due to unpredictable absorption – Useful in the setting of alcohol withdrawal
Lorazepam	2–5 min (IV) 15–30 min (IM)	1–2 mg (IM/IV)	–
Midazolam	2 min (IV) 15 min (IM)	2 mg (IM/IV)	– Higher risk of respiratory depression compared to lorazepam and diazepam
Antipsychotics			
Aripiprazole (atypical antipsychotic)	60 min (IM)	9.75 mg (IM)	– Relatively safe side effect profile
Haloperidol (first-generation antipsychotic)	1–2 min (IV) 30–60 min (IM)	2–5 mg (IM/IV)	– Risk for extrapyramidal symptoms – Higher risk of QTc prolongation, particularly if given IV – IV haloperidol is an off-label route and requires careful monitoring for cardiac arrhythmias if used

	Onset (min)	Initial dose (mg)	Considerations
Olanzapine (atypical antipsychotic)	15–45 min (IM)	10 mg (IM)	– Use with caution when given with benzodiazepines because of increased risk of cardiopulmonary depression – Can cause hypotension
Ziprasidone (atypical antipsychotic)	30–45 min (IM)	20 mg (IM)	– Low risk of QTc prolongation – Not FDA approved for use in the geriatric population

Gillies et al. [17]

Patients who are stratified as low or moderate risk may not require admission for psychiatric treatment, but consultation with a psychiatrist is prudent, especially for moderate-risk patients. Factors arguing for safe discharge of patients with major depressive disorder/unspecified depression include:

- Close follow-up with psychiatric consultant
- Good social support (including someone willing to stay with the patient)
- Absence of high-risk factors mentioned in the above risk factors and history sections

25.9 Other Treatment Modalities

Lifestyle changes, psychotherapy, and pharmacotherapy are effective treatment options for patients with a major depressive episode. The performance of psychotherapy is not appropriate for providers in the emergency setting because of the limited amount of time available. Patients who desire therapy should be referred to providers who can provide these services.

25.9.1 Lifestyle Changes

The following lifestyle changes are efficacious in the treatment of major depressive disorder/unspecified depression:

- Exercise*
- Relaxation therapy*
- Change in diet away from calorie-rich and nutrient-poor foods
- Improved sleep hygiene
  - Including CPAP treatment for individuals with obstructive sleep apnea
- Decreased alcohol intake

*Denotes lifestyle changes that have the best evidence of efficacy [18]

25.9.2 Pharmacotherapy

There is debate whether patients with major depressive disorder/unspecified depression should have pharmacologic therapy initiated in the ED. While over 60% of prescriptions written for antidepressants are written by nonpsychiatrists [18], many emergency providers feel initiation of pharmacotherapy should only be carried out under the direction of a psychiatrist. However, some emergency providers do not have access to an on-call psychiatric specialist and may want to initiate therapy in the emergency setting. When unsure about the need for initiation of pharmacotherapy, there are several decision aids that can be useful. One such aid is the PHQ-9 questionnaire, which uses nine questions to come to a score from 0 to 27. The recommendation is to initiate pharmacotherapy for any patient with a score equal to or greater than 15 [19].

When the decision is made to treat the patient, a second-generation antidepressant should be first line. First-generation antidepressants (tricyclic antidepressants, monoamine oxidase inhibitors) and second-generation antidepressants (selective serotonin reuptake inhibitors, selective norepinephrine reuptake inhibitors, selective serotonin-norepinephrine reuptake inhibitors, and atypical antidepressants) have similar efficacy, but the side effect profile and overall safety relating to possible overdose make second-generation antidepressants a better option. Emergency providers should be familiar with these medications and their side effects; depressed patients may intentionally overdose on these drugs during a suicide attempt.

Classes of antidepressants		
Class	Mechanism of action	Important side effects
Tricyclic antidepressants (TCAs)—amitriptyline, clomipramine, desipramine, doxepin, imipramine, nortriptyline, selegiline, and trimipramine	Blocks action of norepinephrine and serotonin at neural synapses Has some antihistamine and anti-adrenergic effects	• Prolongs QTc • Cardiotoxicity • Arrhythmia • Sedation
Monoamine oxidase inhibitors (MAOIs)—phenelzine, tranylcypromine	Inhibits degradation of monoamine oxidases, which leads to increased levels of neurotransmitters in the neural synapses	• Dietary interaction with tyramine-rich foods (aged cheese, wine) causes uncontrolled hypertension from adrenergic excess • Insomnia
Selective serotonin reuptake inhibitors (SSRIs)—citalopram, escitalopram, fluoxetine, fluvoxamine, paroxetine, and sertraline	Inhibits reuptake of serotonin but not norepinephrine at the neural synapses	• Gastrointestinal upset • Sexual dysfunction • Serotonin syndrome • Increased suicidality in young adults aged 18–24 during initial treatment (generally the first 1–2 months)

Classes of antidepressants		
Class	Mechanism of action	Important side effects
Selective norepinephrine reuptake inhibitors (SNRIs)—desvenlafaxine, duloxetine, levomilnacipran, milnacipran, sibutramine, and venlafaxine	Inhibits the reuptake of norepinephrine at the neural synapses	• Same as SSRIs • Increased blood pressure • Anxiety
Atypical antidepressants—bupropion, mirtazapine, nefazodone, trazodone, vilazodone, and vortioxetine	Variable effects on levels of dopamine, norepinephrine, and serotonin at neural synapses	• Common effects include dry mouth, constipation, and light-headedness • **Trazodone**—priapism and arrhythmias • **Mirtazapine**—arrhythmia • **Nefazodone**—liver dysfunction • **Bupropion**—lowers seizure threshold (avoid in bulimia)

Katon [7]

The side effect profiles of the individual drugs vary within each class and can be tailored by the prescriber to meet specific needs of patients. For example, patients with insomnia may benefit from trazodone due to its sedating effect. The following table contains other examples of important side effects of antidepressants.

Antidepressants and common side effects		
Side effect	Medications	Clinical pearl
Nausea and vomiting	Highest with venlafaxine. Common in multiple antidepressants	• Use extended-release formulation of venlafaxine to reduce nausea • Start at lower doses • Take with food
Diarrhea	Sertraline > paroxetine	• Consider using in patients with constipation
Weight gain	TCAs/MAOIs, mirtazapine > paroxetine	• Consider using in patients with anorexia or unintentional weight loss
Somnolence	Trazodone > mirtazapine	• Use in patients with concurrent insomnia. Dose at night
Dizziness	Venlafaxine > sertraline and duloxetine	• Consider bedtime dosing
Headache	Venlafaxine > bupropion, paroxetine, sertraline, and escitalopram	

Antidepressants and common side effects		
Side effect	Medications	Clinical pearl
Sexual dysfunction	Sertraline > venlafaxine > citalopram > paroxetine Bupropion and mirtazapine do not have this effect	• May require dose reduction or medication switch
Insomnia	Bupropion > sertraline, fluoxetine, paroxetine, and venlafaxine	• Take in the morning
Smoking cessation	Bupropion superior	• Bupropion proven to help patients quit smoking

Katon [7]

Escitalopram and sertraline have been shown in multiple studies to be slightly more efficacious and tolerated than other second-generation antidepressants, making them good first choices [20]. It is important to keep in mind the antidepressant effects of the medications often take several weeks, while the side effects manifest shortly after initiation. Side effects are the most common reason for discontinuation of pharmacotherapy. Thus, patients need to be counseled about common side effects and the importance of continuing treatment as tolerated until the desired effects are achieved.

25.10 Pitfalls in Treating Depressed Patients in the ED

- Failure to ask about a patient's specific plan for committing suicide.
  - A concern of some physicians is if they ask about suicide, there may be an increase in the risk of future suicide attempts. However, this statement has not only been proven to be false, but there is some evidence the opposite might be true [21].
- Patients who state they "only took a few pills" will sometimes be dismissed and not receive a full workup.
  - Patients might be intentionally misleading, and a full evaluation is still necessary.
- Somatic complaints in someone who is depressed are commonly ignored due to providers thinking it is a symptom of their depression.
  - Complaints may hint at a somatic pathology.
  - The opposite is true too; it is important not to ignore someone's depression when they have other pathologies present. This must be addressed prior to discharge.
- Not providing the proper monitoring for a depressed patient.
  - Consider providing a sitter for patients who might harm themselves or others during their ED stay.
- Failure to diagnose major depressive disorder in patients who have terminal conditions.

– Depressed or suicidal thoughts still need to be addressed, and these patients must receive a full psychiatric and safety evaluation.

References

1. Institute of Health Metrics and Evaluation. Global Health Data Exchange (GHDx); 2019. https://vizhub.healthdata.org/gbd-results/?params=gbd-api-2019-permalink/d780dff-be8a381b25e1416884959e88b. Accessed 6 Sept 2022.
2. Georgieva I, Lepping P, Bozev V, et al. Prevalence, new incidence, course, and risk factors of PTSD, depression, anxiety, and panic disorder during the Covid-19 pandemic in 11 countries. Healthcare (Basel). 2021;9(6):664. https://doi.org/10.3390/healthcare9060664.
3. World Health Organization. Depression. https://www.who.int/news-room/fact-sheets/detail/depression. Accessed 6 Sept 2022.
4. Hill T, Jiang Y, Friese CR, Darbes LA, Blazes CK, Zhang X. Analysis of emergency department visits for all reasons by adults with depression in the United States. BMC Emerg Med. 2020;20(1):51. https://doi.org/10.1186/s12873-020-00347-6.
5. Menear M, Doré I, Cloutier AM, et al. The influence of comorbid chronic physical conditions on depression recognition in primary care: a systematic review. J Psychosom Res. 2015;78(4):304–13. https://doi.org/10.1016/J.JPSYCHORES.2014.11.016.
6. Docherty JP. Barriers to the diagnosis of depression in primary care. J Clin Psychiatry. 1997;58(suppl 1):1743. https://www.psychiatrist.com/jcp/depression/barriers-diagnosis-depression-primary-care. Accessed 6 Sept 2022
7. Katon WJ. Epidemiology and treatment of depression in patients with chronic medical illness. Dialogues Clin Neurosci. 2011;13(1):7–23. https://doi.org/10.31887/DCNS.2011.13.1/wkaton.
8. Kessler RC, Berglund P, Demler O, et al. Lifetime prevalence and age-of-onset distributions of DSM-IV disorders in the national comorbidity survey replication. Arch Gen Psychiatry. 2005;62(6):593–602.
9. Mental health for gay and bisexual men | CDC. https://www.cdc.gov/msmhealth/mental-health.htm. Accessed 7 Sept 2022.
10. NIMH. Chronic illness and mental health: recognizing and treating depression. https://www.nimh.nih.gov/health/publications/chronic-illness-mental-health. Accessed 7 Sept 2022.
11. Masango SM, Rataemane ST, Motojesi AA. Suicide and suicide risk factors: a literature review. S Afr Fam Pract. 2008;50(6):25–8. https://doi.org/10.1080/20786204.2008.10873774.
12. Risk and protective factors | Suicide | CDC. https://www.cdc.gov/suicide/factors/index.html. Accessed 7 Sept 2022.
13. American Psychiatric Association. Diagnostic and statistical manual of mental disorders, fifth edition (DSM-5). 5th ed.; 2013.
14. Risk factors, protective factors, and warning signs | AFSP. https://afsp.org/risk-factors-protective-factors-and-warning-signs. Accessed 8 Sept 2022.
15. Hoffman L. Tintinalli's emergency medicine manual: emergency assessment and stabilization of behavioral disorders, 7th ed. McGraw-Hill; 2012.
16. Deal N, Hong M, Matorin A, Shah AA. Stabilization and management of the acutely agitated or psychotic patient. Emerg Med Clin North Am. 2015;33(4):739–52. https://doi.org/10.1016/J.EMC.2015.07.003.
17. Gillies D, Sampson S, Beck A, Rathbone J. Benzodiazepines for psychosis-induced aggression or agitation. Cochrane Database Syst Rev. 2013;2013(4):CD003079. https://doi.org/10.1002/14651858.CD003079.PUB3.
18. Bentley SM, Pagalilauan GL, Simpson SA. Major depression. Med Clin North Am. 2014;98(5):981–1005. https://doi.org/10.1016/J.MCNA.2014.06.013.

19. Kroenke K, Spitzer RL, Williams JBW, Löwe B. The patient health questionnaire somatic, anxiety, and depressive symptom scales: a systematic review. Gen Hosp Psychiatry. 2010;32(4):345–59. https://doi.org/10.1016/J.GENHOSPPSYCH.2010.03.006.
20. Thronson LR, Pagalilauan GL. Psychopharmacology. Med Clin North Am. 2014;98(5):927–58. https://doi.org/10.1016/J.MCNA.2014.06.001.
21. Dazzi T, Gribble R, Wessely S, Fear NT. Does asking about suicide and related behaviours induce suicidal ideation? What is the evidence? Psychol Med. 2014;44:3361. https://doi.org/10.1017/S0033291714001299.

Index

B. K. Desai et al. (eds.), *Primary Care for Emergency Physicians*,
https://doi.org/10.1007/978-3-031-64676-8

MIX
Papier aus verantwortungsvollen Quellen
Paper from responsible sources
FSC® C105338

If you have any concerns about our products,
you can contact us on
ProductSafety@springernature.com

In case Publisher is established outside the EU,
the EU authorized representative is:
Springer Nature Customer Service Center GmbH
Europaplatz 3, 69115 Heidelberg, Germany

Printed by Libri Plureos GmbH
in Hamburg, Germany